Couples and Pregnancy: Welcome, Unwelcome, and In-Between

Couples and Pregnancy: Welcome, Unwelcome, and In-Between has been co-published simultaneously as *Journal of Couples Therapy*, Volume 8, Number 2 1999.

Journal of Couples Therapy Monographic "Separates"

Below is a list of "separates," which in serials librarianship means a special issue simultaneously published as a special journal issue or double-issue and as a "separate" hardbound monograph. (This is a format which we also call a "DocuSerial.")

"Separates" are published because specialized libraries or professionals may wish to purchase a specific thematic issue by itself in a format which can be separately cataloged and shelved, as opposed to purchasing the journal on an on-going basis. Faculty members may also more easily consider a "separate" for classroom adoption.

"Separates" are carefully classified separately with the major book jobbers so that the journal tie-in can be noted on new book order slips to avoid duplicate purchasing.

You may wish to visit Haworth's website at . . .

http://www.haworthpressinc.com

. . . to search our online catalog for complete tables of contents of these separates and related publications.

You may also call 1-800-HAWORTH (outside US/Canada: 607-722-5857), or Fax 1-800-895-0582 (outside US/Canada: 607-771-0012), or e-mail at:

getinfo@haworthpressinc.com

Couples and Pregnancy: Welcome, Unwelcome, and In-Between, edited by Barbara Jo Brothers, MSW, BCSW (Vol. 8, No. 2, 1999). *Gain valuable insight into how pregnancy and birth have a profound psychological effect on the parents' relationship, especially on their experience of intimacy.*

Couples, Trauma, and Catastrophes, edited by Barbara Jo Brothers, MSW, BCSW (Vol. 7, No. 4, 1998). *Helps therapists and counselors working with couples facing major crises and trauma.*

Couples: A Medley of Models, edited by Barbara Jo Brothers, MSW, BCSW (Vol. 7, No. 2/3, 1998). *A wonderful set of authors who illuminate different corners of relationships. This book belongs on your shelf . . . but only after you've read it and loved it. (Derek Paar, PhD, Associate Professor of Psychology, Springfield College, Massachusetts)*

When One Partner Is Willing and the Other Is Not, edited by Barbara Jo Brothers, MSW, BCSW (Vol. 7, No. 1, 1997). *"An engaging variety of insightful perspectives on resistance in couples therapy." (Stan Taubman, DSW, Director of Managed Care, Alameda County Behavioral Health Care Service, Berkeley, California; Author, Ending the Struggle Against Yourself)*

Couples and the Tao of Congruence, edited by Barbara Jo Brothers, MSW, BCSW (Vol. 6, No. 3/4, 1996). *"A library of information linking Virginia Satir's teaching and practice of creative improvement in human relations and the Tao of Congruence. . . .A stimulating reader." (Josephine A. Bates, DSW, BD, retired mental health researcher and family counselor, Lake Preston, South Dakota)*

Couples and Change, edited by Barbara Jo Brothers, MSW, BCSW (Vol. 6, No. 1/2, 1996). *This enlightening book presents readers with Satir's observations–observations that show the difference between thinking with systems in mind and thinking linearly–of process, interrelatedness, and attitudes.*

Couples and Countertransference, edited by Barbara Jo Brothers, MSW, BCSW (Vol. 5, No. 3, 1995). *"I would recommend this book to beginning and advanced couple therapists as well as to social workers and psychologists. . . . This book is a wealth of information." (International Transactional Analysis Association.)*

Couples: Building Bridges, edited by Barbara Jo Brothers, MSW, BCSW (Vol. 5, No. 4, 1996.) *"This work should be included in the library of anyone considering to be a therapist or who is one or who is fascinated by the terminology and conceptualizations which the study of marriage utilizes." (Irv Loev, PhD, MSW-ACP, LPC, LMFT, private practitioner)*

Power and Partnering, edited by Barbara Jo Brothers, MSW, BCSW (Vol. 5, No. 1/2, 1995). *"Appeals to therapists and lay people who find themselves drawn to the works of Virginia Satir and Carl Jung. Includes stories and research data satisfying the tastes of both left- and right-brained readers." (Virginia O. Felder, ThM, Licensed Marriage and Family Therapist, private practice, Atlanta, Georgia)*

Surpassing Threats and Rewards: Newer Plateaus for Couples and Coupling, edited by Barbara Jo Brothers, MSW, BCSW (Vol. 4, No. 3/4, 1995). *Explores the dynamics of discord, rejection, and blame in the coupling process and provides practical information to help readers understand marital dissatisfaction and how this dissatisfaction manifests itself in relationships.*

Attraction and Attachment: Understanding Styles of Relationships, edited by Barbara Jo Brothers, MSW, BCSW (Vol. 4, No. 1/2, 1994). *"Ideas on working effectively with couples. . . . I strongly recommend this book for those who want to have a better understanding of the complex dynamics of couples and couples therapy." (Gilbert J. Greene, PhD, ACSW, Associate Professor, College of Social Work, The Ohio State University)*

Peace, War, and Mental Health: Couples Therapists Look at the Dynamics, edited by Barbara Jo Brothers, MSW, BCSW (Vol. 3, No. 4, 1993). *Discover how issues of world war and peace relate to the dynamics of couples therapy in this thought-provoking book.*

Couples Therapy, Multiple Perspectives: In Search of Universal Threads, edited by Barbara Jo Brothers, MSW, BCSW (Vol. 3, No. 2/3, 1993). *"A very sizeable team of couples therapists has scoured the countryside in search of the most effective methods for helping couples improve their relationships. . . . The bibliographies are a treasury of worthwhile references." (John F. Sullivan, EdS, Marriage and Family Counselor in Private Practice, Newburgh, New York)*

Spirituality and Couples: Heart and Soul in the Therapy Process, edited by Barbara Jo Brothers, MSW, BCSW (Vol. 3, No. 1, 1993). *"Provides an array of reflections particularly for therapists beginning to address spirituality in the therapeutic process." (Journal of Family Psychotherapy)*

Equal Partnering: A Feminine Perspective, edited by Barbara Jo Brothers, MSW, BCSW (Vol. 2, No. 4, 1992). *Designed to help couples, married or not, understand how to achieve a balanced, equal partnership.*

Coupling . . . What Makes Permanence?, edited by Barbara Jo Brothers, MSW, BCSW (Vol. 2, No. 3, 1991). *"Explores what it is that makes for a relationship in which each partner can grow and develop while remaining attached to another." (The British Journal of Psychiatry)*

Virginia Satir: Foundational Ideas, edited by Barbara Jo Brothers, MSW, BCSW (Vol. 2, No. 1/2, 1991). *"The most thorough conglomeration of her ideas available today. Done in the intimate, yet clear fashion you would expect from Satir herself. . . . Well worth getting your hands damp to pick up this unique collection." (Journal of Family Psychotherapy)*

Intimate Autonomy: Autonomous Intimacy, edited by Barbara Jo Brothers, MSW, BCSW (Vol. 1, No. 3/4, 1991). *"A fine collection of chapters on one of the most difficult of human tasks–getting close enough to another to share the warmth and benefits of that closeness without losing what is precious in our separations." (Howard Halpern, PhD, Author, How to Break Your Addiction to a Person)*

Couples on Coupling, edited by Barbara Jo Brothers, MSW, BCSW (Vol. 1, No. 2, 1990). *"A variety of lenses through which to view relationships, each providing a different angle for seeing patterns, strengths, and problems and for gaining insight into a given couple system." (Suzanne Imes, PhD, Clinical Psychologist, Private Practice, Atlanta, Georgia; Adjunct Assistant Professor of Psychology, Georgia State University)*

Couples and pregnancy

Couples and Pregnancy: Welcome, Unwelcome, and In-Between has been co-published simultaneously as *Journal of Couples Therapy,* Volume 8, Number 2 1999.

The development, preparation, and publication of this work has been undertaken with great care. However, the publisher, employees, editors, and agents of The Haworth Press and all imprints of The Haworth Press, Inc., including The Haworth Medical Press® and Pharmaceutical Products Press®, are not responsible for any errors contained herein or for consequences that may ensue from use of materials or information contained in this work. Opinions expressed by the author(s) are not necessarily those of The Haworth Press, Inc.

The Haworth Press, Inc., 10 Alice Street, Binghamton, NY 13904-1580 USA

Cover design by Thomas J. Mayshock Jr.

Library of Congress Cataloging-in-Publication Data

Couples and pregnancy: welcome, unwelcome, and in-between/Barbara Jo Brothers, editor.
    p. cm.
    "Has been co-published simultaneously as Journal of couples therapy, Volume 8, Number 2, 1999."
    Includes bibliographical references and index.
    ISBN 0-7890-0787-8 (alk. paper).–ISBN 0-7890-0822-X (pbk.: alk. paper)
    1. Marital psychotherapy. 2. Interpersonal relations. 3. Pregnancy Miscellanea. I. Brothers, Barbara Jo, 1940- . II. Journal of couples therapy.
RC488.5.C64317 1999
616.89'156–dc21
                                                          99-38461
                                                           CIP

Couples and Pregnancy: Welcome, Unwelcome, and In-Between

Barbara Jo Brothers
Editor

Couples and Pregnancy: Welcome, Unwelcome, and In-Between has been co-published simultaneously as *Journal of Couples Therapy*, Volume 8, Number 2 1999.

The Haworth Press, Inc.
New York • London • Oxford

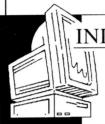

INDEXING & ABSTRACTING

Contributions to this publication are selectively indexed or abstracted in print, electronic, online, or CD-ROM version(s) of the reference tools and information services listed below. This list is current as of the copyright date of this publication. See the end of this section for additional notes.

- *Abstracts of Research in Pastoral Care & Counseling*

- *BUBL Information Service: An Internet-Based Information Service for the UK Higher Education Community <URL:http://bubl.ac.uk>*

- *CNPIEC Reference Guide: Chinese Directory of Foreign Periodicals*

- *Family Studies Database (online and CD/ROM)*

- *Family Violence & Sexual Assault Bulletin*

- *Mental Health Abstracts (online through DIALOG)*

- *Referativnyi Zhurnal (Abstracts Journal of the All-Russian Institute of Scientific and Technical Information)*

- *Social Planning/Policy & Development Abstracts (SOPODA)*

- *Social Work Abstracts*

- *Sociological Abstracts (SA)*

- *Studies on Women Abstracts*

- *Violence and Abuse Abstracts: A Review of Current Literature on Interpersonal Violence (VAA)*

(continued)

*Special Bibliographic Notes related to special journal issues
(separates) and indexing/abstracting:*

- indexing/abstracting services in this list will also cover material in any "separate" that is co-published simultaneously with Haworth's special thematic journal issue or DocuSerial. Indexing/abstracting usually covers material at the article/chapter level.
- monographic co-editions are intended for either non-subscribers or libraries which intend to purchase a second copy for their circulating collections.
- monographic co-editions are reported to all jobbers/wholesalers/approval plans. The source journal is listed as the "series" to assist the prevention of duplicate purchasing in the same manner utilized for books-in-series.
- to facilitate user/access services all indexing/abstracting services are encouraged to utilize the co-indexing entry note indicated at the bottom of the first page of each article/chapter/contribution.
- this is intended to assist a library user of any reference tool (whether print, electronic, online, or CD-ROM) to locate the monographic version if the library has purchased this version but not a subscription to the source journal.
- individual articles/chapters in any Haworth publication are also available through the Haworth Document Delivery Service (HDDS).

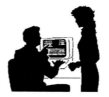

Couples and Pregnancy: Welcome, Unwelcome, and In-Between

CONTENTS

ABOUT THE EDITOR

Barbara Jo Brothers, MSW, BCD, a Diplomate in Clinical Social Work, National Association of Social Workers, is in private practice in New Orleans. She received her BA from the University of Texas and her MSW from Tulane University, where she is currently on the faculty. She was Editor of *The Newsletter of the American Academy of Psychotherapists* from 1976 to 1985, and was Associate Editor of *Voices: The Art and Science of Psychotherapy* from 1979 to 1989. She has 30 years of experience, in both the public and private sectors, helping people to form skills that will enable them to connect emotionally. The author of numerous articles and book chapters on authenticity in human relating, she has advocated healthy, congruent communication that builds intimacy as opposed to destructive, incongruent communication which blocks intimacy. In addition to her many years of direct work with couples and families, Ms. Brothers has led numerous workshops on teaching communication in families and has also played an integral role in the development of training programs in family therapy for mental health workers throughout the Louisiana state mental health system. She is a board member of the Institute for International Connections, a non-profit organization for cross-cultural professional development focused on training and cross-cultural exchange with psychotherapists in Russia, republics once part of what used to be the Soviet Union, and other Eastern European countries.

"We Are Only Activators"–
Virginia Satir
and the Mystery of Human Life:
A Reflection

Barbara Jo Brothers

SUMMARY. Edited transcription of three lectures, given by Virginia Satir, on the same topic, but presented in three different ways. Lectures were each a part of a month-long seminar given in 1981, 1982, and 1983 during module I of the Avanta Process Community Meetings in Crested Butte, Colorado. *[Article copies available for a fee from The Haworth Document Delivery Service: 1-800-342-9678. E-mail address: getinfo@haworthpressinc.com <Website: http://www.haworthpressinc.com>]*

KEYWORDS. Manifestation of Life Force, activators versus creators

On many occasions, Virginia Satir spoke of various facets of our human nature . . . our uniqueness, yet our unwearying similarity; our differences–yet our passion for union and harmony. No matter the subject specifically targeted, Virginia always found it necessary to point out–then to simply admire the mystery of our unique origination. Over and over again she would repeat: "We are not creators of life; we are only activators."

She wanted to make clear the implications and ramifications of this vital fact. It was her belief that, were this widely accepted, child-rearing would proceed very differently. In understanding that we are each a unique man-

---

Printed with permission of Avanta: The Virginia Satir Network, 2104 S.W. 152nd Street, #2, Burien, WA 98166.

[Haworth co-indexing entry note]: "'We Are Only Activators'–Virginia Satir and the Mystery of Human Life: A Reflection." Brothers, Barbara Jo. Co-published simultaneously in *Journal of Couples Therapy* (The Haworth Press, Inc.) Vol. 8, No. 2, 1999, pp. 1-5; and: *Couples and Pregnancy: Welcome, Unwelcome, and In-Between* (ed: Barbara Jo Brothers) The Haworth Press, Inc., 1999, pp. 1-5.

ifestation of Life, we would spare ourselves much of the unnecessary anguish and stubborn pain inherent in individuals trying to fit into molds and/or trying to fit others into molds. We would honor both our own personhood and that of others.

I would invite you now to read several excerpts from Virginia's Avanta Process Community Meetings, given at Crested Butte, Colorado seminars, dealing with the same topic. You will notice that Virginia in each successive year repeats the fact: "we are only activators." She is not merely "repeating herself." She is seeking to impress upon her hearers and readers–upon the entire world–a fact which, if taken seriously, would indeed bring about several happy revolutions: this fact is the paradoxical uniqueness and sameness of the sacred human person.

In the August 1981 meeting, Virginia is emphasizing our equality in value and worth, building a base for development of self-esteem, crucial to emotional growth:

> . . . So the world is changing here, giving out some new possibilities . . . the beginnings of another view of how we can look at people . . . we saw Abe Maslow . . . and Rollo May [talking about] the definition of a relationship as one of equality. Now that sounds peculiar, because how can everybody be equal? You know, some are tall, some are short, some . . .
>
> Now what that really meant is that our navels are equal in the sense that we all came the same way. This had to do with value and worth, that people are of value. And they equal each other in value and manifestation of life force. If we really believe what we are told on the theological level that we are made in the image or likenesses of the creator, how can we be unequal? . . . So we began to say person equals person because they have navels and because they are manifestations of self-worth.
>
> Now, this was so new [it] brought not only discovery, at first it [also] brought dismay. How could I, a four-year-old, feel equal to my mother, a 44-year-old? How could I, a student, feel equal to my professor? You didn't have the same amounts of knowledge or the same age. [Equality is not about those factors. It is about this:] you are a manifestation of life-force, This was discovery, and another discovery in relation to that is that a person is unique. Every person is a combination of sameness and differentness in relation to every other person. So it isn't: if you love me we'll be the same and if you don't love, you'll be different. It is: the genuine, basic nature of the human being is a combination of sameness and differentness.
>
> That meant then, that there were no duplicates of people . . . We are each unique; the *sperm and the egg . . . no human being to date has been able to create life. They can activate it, but they can't create it.*

Nobody has created a sperm, nobody has created an ovum. That still remains a secret of the universe.

So, then we must know that since we don't create anything, we only activate it–it's already created–we are all part of the same life-force and energy that gets activated in our particular context. Each individual gets activated however they do, and move up and move down [in the current of life]. That asks us to look at human life in quite a different way, with both reverence and a sacredness and with a reality that we haven't been able to do before. Also tremendous hope [comes with] that.

[Many other ideas come in here.] How to discover uniqueness? How does the harmony come to unity [around] opposites? Or you can put it, the unity between what is the opposite and what is the same–the harmony between the two. How do we put dark and light together, how do we put men and women together, how do we put short and tall together, how do we put different belief systems together, how do we live in a place where people believe differently, and still can have a harmony?

Now we are in the process of discovery . . . [uniqueness and sameness, differences with harmony.] (1981, p. 68-71)

In her lecture at the 1982 Meeting, Virginia points out our role as co-directors, rather than creators, of our lives:

. . . There is another piece; once we get to it another absolutely fantastic awareness develops: you think you created your children.

You did not. All you did was activate the ingredients so that life could happen.

You did not create anything. You only activated the opportunity–on purpose or otherwise. So we do not create life; we do not create it at all. It is already created. Once we get there [to that awareness], we know absolutely that we are spiritual beings. No one, to date, has been able to create life. It is created. So now we come into our spiritual base. It does not necessarily have to be with any religion, [though] it could. Life is all here; we just keep having it formed and reformed. And there are three words I want to give you that fit here and that are very dear to me: self, eggs and seeds. Once we see what is right in front of our noses–that we are spiritual beings tuning in and getting life from this planet–then we can begin to be co-creators of how we use that life. Co-directors of how we use that life. Let us never mix up [and think] that we are the creators of our life. We are the co-directors of how it goes, and as such we use the perceptions that we have to direct our life.

. . . The life force, there is no end and no beginning; it is just there. If we were to think of it as an ongoing river, every once in a while something comes together like a fountain–which is one of us–takes that life force and makes all kinds of splashes. Because we were born little, we will splash in accordance to what we were taught, not in terms of how we could splash in many different ways. So here is the underpinnings: we activate the life-force, we co-direct how things are going to happen; we do not create ourselves. Now that is a very great difference from having a picture of "how you should be" and cutting off or hiding that which does not fit. Totally different approach. So you can see that anything about child-rearing that is based on this [concept of spirituality] is going to lead to a totally different result than when based on this [the threat/reward approach]. (1994, p. 6-7)

In the 1983 Meeting, Virginia points again to our spiritual base:

. . . we began suddenly to be aware that *no human being creates life.* There's no way, there is no way to create life. No one has been able to create an egg and sperm that can make a human being. That's there, that's a given. So what we do is we *activate* life, we activate that. And by a sperm and egg coming together–which is the original plan which we had nothing to do with–then life comes. You had nothing to do with how you were activated except in maybe an esoteric sense. You get activated and then there's a whole program there for you. You didn't make it. No scientist sat down at the drawing board to figure out a person, that was there.

Now then, we had to face the fact, where do we get created? That's our spiritual base. That is already there and I look at it as a river that goes on all the time. That's the basis of ourselves, the spiritual base, that which makes it possible for the egg and sperm to come together. And that can or can not be religious in my terms. You all know what I'm talking about and I think many people know that too. So what we are in–this coming together, the sperm and egg, [via] our parents through their genitals and through the internal, beautiful engineering that they have to carry this egg and sperm, and then we come up like a fountain. And then we do the same thing [concerning the genitals and "the internal, beautiful engineering"] and some more fountains are . . . [made] And each one of us becomes a co-creator after we get here, based upon this spiritual [fact]. (1992, p. 10-11)

We come into this world with both guaranteed similarities and guaranteed variation. From Virginia Satir's way of thinking, each one of us is a unique creation and manifestation of the Life Force–and deserving of a corresponding measure of respect.

REFERENCES

Brothers, B. J. (Ed.) (1992). Virginia Satir's Spirituality, *Spirituality and Couples: Heart and Soul in the Therapy Process*. Binghamton, NY: The Haworth Press, Inc.
Brothers, B.J. (1994) From Virginia Satir: Beyond the Threat/Reward Model. *Surpassing Threats and Rewards*. Binghamton, NY: The Haworth Press, Inc.
Satir, V. (1981). Virginia Satir at the University of Utah. Unpublished transcript.

Pregnancy, Intimacy,
and the Family Constitution

Andrew I. Schwebel

SUMMARY. The psychological effects of pregnancy and birth have a profound effect on the parents' relationship, especially on their experience of intimacy. The nature of the impact on the couple depends on the developmental stage of each parent and the couple's ability to adapt to new circumstances. Three developmental stages are described and the "family constitution" is presented as the body of goals, rules and roles that governs the behavior of the family and effectively managing the constitution is introduced and applied to two sets of circumstances related to pregnancy. Finally, the implications of the above concepts for therapists and counselors are delineated. [*Article copies available for a fee from The Haworth Document Delivery Service: 1-800-342-9678. E-mail address: getinfo@haworthpressinc.com <Website: http://www.haworthpressinc.com>]*

KEYWORD. Pregnancy, intimacy, developmental stages

Andrew I. Schwebel: February 5, 1943-June 4, 1996

Between the time of writing this article and its publication, Andrew Schwebel died. We regret that we will be receiving no more such well-written, practical-approach articles from him.

Dr. Schwebel's father, Dr. Milton Schwebel, is editor of *Peace and Conflict: Journal of Peace Psychology–The Journal of the Division of Peace Psychology of the American Psychological Association.* He requested that publication continue as planned. Correspondence about this article should be sent to Milton Schwebel, Graduate School of Applied and Professional Psychology, Rutgers University, Piscataway, NJ 08855-0819.

[Haworth co-indexing entry note]: "Pregnancy, Intimacy, and the Family Constitution." Schwebel, Andrew I. Co-published simultaneously in *Journal of Couples Therapy* (The Haworth Press, Inc.) Vol. 8, No. 2, 1999, pp. 7-16; and: *Couples and Pregnancy: Welcome, Unwelcome, and In-Between* (ed: Barbara Jo Brothers) The Haworth Press, Inc., 1999, pp. 7-16. Single or multiple copies of this article are available for a fee from The Haworth Document Delivery Service [1-800-342-9678, 9:00 a.m. - 5:00 p.m. (EST). E-mail address: getinfo@haworthpressinc.com].

When the act of sexual intercourse results in conception and birth, it produces concrete biological effects in the form of offspring. By contrast, the psychological effects resulting from pregnancy and birth are much less obvious. However, these effects are profound in the life of partners in an ongoing relationship.

This article focuses on some of these psychological effects and especially on the impact of pregnancy and birth on a couple's experience of intimacy. The impact can be positive or negative. Among the factors central to whether pregnancy and birth enhance a couple's intimacy, or detract from it, are the following: (1) the developmental stage of each parent and (2) the ability of a couple to establish and adjust in response to changes they face in their relationship as they become parents.

Below I introduce a three-stage model of an individual's ability to be intimate and then discuss the concept of the "family constitution," which concretizes the method by which couples adjust to change, regulate their shared lives, and cope with new developments, such as pregnancy. Following that, I discuss clinical applications of this model.

THREE DEVELOPMENTAL STAGES

There are many informative and pragmatically useful perspectives on the development of the individual across the life span including Erikson (1980), Levinson (1978) on men, and Gilligan (1982) and Roberts and Newton (1987) on women. For present purposes, however, we will use a simple three stage model of an individual's capacity for intimacy that focuses on only one factor: the person's capacity to be a healthy, "giving" partner in a family relationship.

In stage one, the individual values "my personal freedom and independence. I don't want or need a permanent relationship with another person. I can satisfy all my needs without that." In stage two the person values "a permanent relationship with another adult. I yearn for that kind of interdependence where I'll help satisfy my partner's needs and my partner will help satisfy mine." Finally, in stage three, the individual values "more than an interdependent relationship, I want to care for and nurture a child who is fully dependent upon my spouse and me. I don't ask for anything in return, although I'm sure I'll receive much emotional gratification."

Many people attempt to establish couple relationships without reaching stage two. The result is self-centered, competitive interactions. Of those who reach stage two, some never advance to stage three. Those who do move from a focus on self-gratification to a focus on the gratification of another can advance to stages two and three. Taken as a whole, the three stages represent steps in a path that individuals follow in a personal, social and an evolutionary course of development. People advance from merely seeking personal gratification toward forming nurturing relationships with another individual and finally toward a relationship that sustains the species.

An individual's personal development–his or her capacity for intimacy–is a factor that will influence the couple's relationship during and after pregnancy. If both members of the dyad have reached the third stage by the time the pregnancy has begun, they will be able to avoid many individual development-related problems. If, however, one or both members are frozen at the stage of wanting the relationship solely to fulfill ego-centric needs for self-gratification, such as gaining financial advantage, sexual convenience, or to establish a dependency status, the partners will inevitably experience serious problems and may not be able to adjust successfully to the pregnancy and baby.

THE FAMILY CONSTITUTION

To more fully comprehend the changes in the quality of a couple's relation-ship during pregnancy, we need to understand how they modified their rela-tionship in response to the new conditions; i.e., how successful they were in consciously transforming the way of life of a two-adult couple to that of the two-adult/pregnant couple. Conditions and circumstances change with preg-nancy: As the wife's body changes, she may endure considerable discomfort limiting her ability to perform some of the activities she was accustomed to doing. The husband's psyche is also undergoing modification as a consequence of changes in his view of himself and his future, and of observed changes in his wife. How the partners react and what actions they take to modify their way of life will determine their success in navigating these changing seas.

I have written elsewhere about the construct of the "family constitution" which describes the entire set of unwritten and ever-changing rules that govern life between partners and in families (Schwebel & Fine, 1992, 1994). A couple's family constitution spells out broad issues in their relationship, such as how they should communicate, share resources and responsibilities, make decisions, and interact with other people. The family constitution also delineates specific policies and procedures, ranging from who is responsible for preparing dinner on a Saturday night to how the toothpaste tube should be squeezed.

Although family members are not usually aware of the fact that they have a family constitution, in actuality they played a key role in shaping it. Further-more, they remain actively involved in the process of directing changes in it so that it helps them live comfortably as members of the couple and family unit.

HOW THE FAMILY CONSTITUTION CHANGES

Most rules are added to the family constitution or modified in two ways: (1) through discussion between the partners as they plan future activities or solve problems, and (2) through precedent. In the latter case, one partner behaves in a particular way and, experiencing no negative feedback from the other partner, establishes, by precedent, that a particular behavior is acceptable in the relationship. The rule governing the behavior becomes part of the family constitution.

Change in the constitution begins early after conception. The moment the couple learns that the pregnancy test is positive, they begin to experience a change in consciousness as they realize their newly acquired opportunity for fulfillment and growth. Couples who understand that successful marriage requires the establishment of mutually acceptable family goals are at an advantage when pregnancy occurs, because they realize that new goals now have to be written. These goals will now encompass the additional member of the family, as the husband and wife begin to think about the offspring's future, as well as of the future of their family as an entity.

Besides goals, they must rewrite their roles and responsibilities: Some tasks borne by the wife up to this point may have to be carried by the husband, and vice versa. Entirely new roles, in particular those in child care (e.g., feeding, diapering, bathing, stimulating, night-tending) must be identified and assigned.

Those who are personally ready to move to stage three *and* have been guided up to this point by consciously derived constitutions will have little if any difficulty in amending their agreements in accord with the new realities. The months of pregnancy and the early years of child care will form a seamless path. The transformation of the constitution from one made for a couple to one for a family will have few, if any, serious problems.

This is not to suggest "romance made in heaven." On the contrary, conflict is inevitable. However, those who are accustomed to amend their constitution in the face of new conditions will have worked out equitable assignments and, in any case, will have methods to address and resolve differences. Instead of power plays, resentment and hostile silence or paybacks, they will have an available repertoire of peaceful conflict resolution methods. Living this way, confident in their ability to work out problems to their mutual satisfaction, their relationship will be strengthened.

INTIMACY IN PREGNANCY

A pregnancy might suggest that the soon-to-appear new family member will have a dulling effect on intimacy. On the contrary, new circumstances can elicit a deeper form of closeness. Two adults who confront and transcend new and complex issues associated with pregnancy and child-rearing will see each other in a more mature light. Not only is the spouse "the mother/father of my child" but also the partner with whom the problems of the new stage are being surmounted. Like those who have endured a crisis together, such as being lost in a forest and finding a way out, the bond is stronger than before.

Pregnancy intertwines two people as marriage cannot. Spouses who divorce have nothing that still tie them together but memories. Since most of these, especially the more recent ones, are unhappy, the ties are quickly shattered. However, once the two have a child in common, the tie between the spouses is a permanent one. Even after divorce, they cannot alter the fact that the former spouse will forever be the other parent of their child, and they must interact with the spouse if they both are to have a connection with their child, for example, in respect to visitation rights, birthdays, vacations and the like.

For spouses who have rewritten their constitution in health-promoting ways, the intertwining naturally tightens the bond between them. This, in turn, deepens their level of intimacy, be it in the spiritual, companionship, or sexual form. Still lovers, they are now partners in a more complex, cooperative effort than any they had experienced before. They are partners in bringing a pregnancy to a successful conclusion. Couples whose constitution calls for joint efforts and equal participation, do not equate the post-conception nine months as "feminine business." Both parties become students of the intricacies of fetal development, the pregnancy experience, and labor and delivery. In some cases both parties participate in the delivery. "Doing it together" could be a theme song not only about the sexual act that begins it all but also about the excitement at the life stirring within the womb, their concern about the delivery, their joint involvement in infant care, and the life of the little one forever thereafter.

Spouses who are at an earlier level of individual development, motivated to have a baby but too egocentric to nurture it, need professional help. Because the spouses are frozen at an earlier stage, they do not readily have access to the motivation and skills necessary to write a health-promoting revision of their family constitution. They go through a period of intra- and inter-individual struggle. More than a century ago in his classic play, "The Doll's House," Henrik Ibsen revealed the unhappy outcome when immature adults become parents. During a crisis, when Nora discovered that she was just a doll, a play thing to her banker husband who wants her unchanged, she realizes that she will not be fit to be a wife and mother until she, herself, becomes an adult. She walks out of her home, leaving behind her children and desperately pleading husband, with a vague promise that she would return when she had become a person in her own right.

We can only speculate about how many marriages have floundered on those same rocks, usually without either spouse benefitting from Nora's insights. Usually one or both spouses are frozen at an early developmental stage, and when life becomes difficult–due to any variety of factors such as sleep deprivation from caring for a baby, financial demands, or the stress of new roles–they find excuses to escape physically or psychologically. They are unable to adjust to the new circumstances.

THE BASIC PRINCIPLE
OF EFFECTIVELY MANAGING THE CONSTITUTION

The basic principle is that successful marriage and parenting require intelligent, cooperative planning. It is true that some couples manage to get by without pre-pregnancy planning and even without thoughtful planning at all. In some cases of this kind, the spouses come to grips with problems only as and when they encounter them. Then they deal with them as a couple. In other cases, the two partners do not talk about problems at all. Instead, when problems arise, one acts to deal with it and the other reacts, so there is no "putting two heads together," no coordination, not even of the impromptu kind. In both of these cases, problem solving effectiveness is diminished by a weak constitution. With their constitutions, they are not able to bring their full, combined resources to bear upon addressing the new circumstances. To move past this block, they must make changes by redefining the previously-established (and now outdated) goals, rules and roles in their constitution.

By contrast, effective couples sit down and discuss how they have been living their lives, and how they must now look ahead and modify their schedules, household chore-management, vacations, social life and career schedules–all of which are necessary steps in the process of consciously rewriting the constitution to meet the new demands of life. As in other important aspects of human functioning, conscious, deliberate thinking and careful scheduling and strategizing give order, stability and security to life without diminishing opportunities for spontaneity.

The principle of managing the family constitution remains constant in varied circumstances. Below we consider its applicability in two different sets of circumstances related to pregnancy: first, whether the pregnancy is planned or unplanned; second whether it is the first or second pregnancy.

Planned or Unplanned. The family constitution is relevant in both planned or unplanned pregnancies. Let us assume that in both instances the couples already have a consciously developed constitution. The parties are clear about their goals as a unit and as individuals. They have defined their rules of behavior and their household roles, and have a repertoire of conflict resolution procedures. In the case of the planned pregnancy, chances are the two already will have begun the process of amending the constitution even before conception. In contrast, the couple confronted with an unplanned pregnancy will start from scratch only after the surprise/shock and the realization of its implications set in. They are at an initial disadvantage but, nonetheless, have ample opportunity to catch up and prepare themselves for changed conditions.

Some couples with unplanned pregnancies find the condition unwelcome and yet will not have an abortion. For a successful family outcome, they will have to amend their constitution in ways that enable the spouses to redefine their individual and family goals. Career plans may have to be modified, the completion of an educational program temporarily postponed, the purchase of a new car delayed. The important objective at this moment is to accommodate to the unwanted situation in such ways that leave the partners without ambivalence in their feelings toward their forthcoming offspring.

First, Second or Later Born Children. Therapists often have to correct the popular belief that a second and subsequent pregnancies, and the infants born from them, are easily taken in stride because of the experience acquired during the first or earlier ones. It is true that as "veteran" couples they can anticipate the progress of the pregnancy. Unfortunately, however, they may infer that child-care experiences with the first give them the same advantage in planning child-care for the second child. They may be unaware of three fundamental principles:

1. Demands on the parents more than double as they must accommodate to the needs of an additional child. The requisite effort is also greater because the children will be at different developmental stages. The consequent fatigue and the possible philosophical differences between the parents in the mode of child care and discipline can give rise to conflict between them.

2. The personality and attentional needs of the first are not necessarily predictive of those features in the second child. The second one may be more, much more, less, or much less demanding of attention. Some of the difference, e.g., that due to temperament (Chess & Thomas, 1987), may even be evident during pregnancy, with one fetus relatively passive and another moving and kicking wildly. Furthermore, the reactions of each of the parents to each child may be different, setting off a circular effect with the respective child. For example, one child looks like a likable (or unlikable) sibling, or resembles those in one's own or the spouse's family, giving rise, in either case, to a positive or negative reaction in the parent at a low level of consciousness.

3. When the first child appears on the scene, the family complex of relationships increases in quantity from one (H<>W) to four (H<>W, H<>1st, W<>1st, (circle of H,W,1st)). With the second child, the quantity of relationships goes from four to nine: The four above plus these five (H<>2nd, W<>2nd, 1st<>2nd, (circle of HW2nd, and HW1st2nd)). The possibility of enriched loving relationships increases, but so, too, does the possibility of new problems due to lesser parental time avail-

able to devote to the first child and the likelihood of competition between siblings.

Clear-headed and well-informed anticipation of what lies ahead is just as vital for parents in their adjustment to the second pregnancy as to the first. The couple must modify the family constitution as it relates to parental roles and rules of attending to children's physical and psychological needs. The constitution must be altered in order to plan matters related to education and discipline. The couple also must safeguard the intimacy in their relationship, for the sake of the children as well as themselves.

IMPLICATIONS FOR THERAPISTS, COUNSELORS AND OTHER HELP-GIVERS

It is important that professionals working with couples and families coping with pregnancy and childbirth have a thorough understanding of the following: the three stages of individual development in the capacity for intimacy, the family constitution (including the modes of amending and rewriting it), and the varied conditions under which a pregnancy occurs (i.e., planned or unplanned; the first or subsequent pregnancy). Professionals must also be skilled in applying their knowledge. In their work with couples, they need to have experience, preferably under supervision or, at least, through self-monitoring by use of video recordings, in using these concepts. To guard against counselor/therapist bias and personal involvement (counter-transference), it is important for help-givers to apply these concepts to their own personal development and relationships.

The three sets of knowledge should be integrated. Knowing only about individual development does not help with matters related to the family constitution. With the latter knowledge, one can obtain meaningful information about how the partners typically interact when encountering changed circumstances, such as those represented by a pregnancy, i.e., whether they change their behavior as individuals and/or as a couple, and if so, in what direction and with what effect. Still, to be optimally helpful, even that knowledge is insufficient because it does not inform us of the circumstances of the pregnancy.

To illustrate the above points, consider the case of Bill and Kate Davis who come to the counselor (C) because they are having conflict over her pregnancy. Bill says that his mother feels strongly that Kate should quit her job after the first trimester, and he concurs. But he is actually troubled over having his life disrupted by having to do more work around the house than before because Kate is often tired at the end of the day. Kate refuses to quit her job. C is unaware of the factors that relate to intimacy during pregnancy.

C decides to focus on the need for compromise; to get Bill's current and future load more acceptable to him, and perhaps even reduced through some means. C does not realize that Bill is self-centered, in the first stage of individual development and incapable of a close relationship at this time. C is attempting to arrive at a solution to this problem without examining critical factors and addressing key questions such as the following:

Individual Capacity for Intimacy

- What is Kate's developmental stage in terms of intimacy?
- What is Bill's developmental stage in terms of intimacy?

Pregnancy

- Was this a planned pregnancy?
- Did Bill want a child as much as Kate did?
- Did they discuss and anticipate the changes in their lives that the pregnancy and a child would require? If so, how realistic an appraisal did they make? Did Bill participate actively in the appraisal? Did he clearly comprehend the consequences *for him* of the pregnancy?

Family Constitution

- Are they aware of their family constitution?
- If not, are they aware of how they typically confront changed circumstances in the past?
- How do they cope with conflict: Through denial, avoidance, unilateral decision-making, impulsive reflex action, physical power, discussion, rational decision-making, mediation?

We want all this information from Bill and Kate. We also want to know how the decision to have a baby occurred. If the pregnancy was planned, to what extent were Kate, Bill, and Bill's mother involved in the decision? What is the role of each partner's parents in the family constitution? What was Bill's attitude about having a child before they were married, afterward and when the decision was made? What level of foresight did Bill have before the pregnancy of the effects on their respective domestic work schedules?

It would be valuable to know how they handled conflict in the past, possibly by focusing on recent examples. Reviewing these examples, how was each resolved? What were the respective partners' degree of satisfaction with the resolutions? Did they use the same mode of conflict resolution each time? If not, how did the methods differ? What is their typical way of resolving conflicts? Who plays what roles in the process? During the course of their relationship, have they changed their mode of dealing with conflict?

C's probing is not only to help them resolve their current conflict but also to heighten their awareness of the following:

- Their respective levels of development in their capacity for intimate relationships.
- Their mode(s) of addressing (or ignoring) change and conflict and of coping with them.
- The possibility of improving each of the above.

As professionals, we can ill-afford to ignore or neglect any information vital to understanding and assisting couples grappling with problems evoked by pregnancy and childbirth. Knowledge and skill in use of the concepts of individual development, the family constitution and the conditions of pregnancy are professional imperatives.

REFERENCES

Chess, S. & Thomas, A. (1987). *Know your child.* New York: Basic Books.

Erikson, E. (1980). *Identity and the life cycle.* N.Y.: Norton.

Gilligan, C. (1982). *In a different voice.* Cambridge: Harvard University Press.

Levinson, D. (1978). *Seasons of a man's life.* N.Y.: Ballantine.

Roberts, P. & Newton, P. M. (1987). Levinsonian studies of women's adult development. *Psychology and Aging,* 2(2), 154-163.

Schwebel, A.I. & Fine, M.A. (1992). Cognitive-behavioral family therapy. *Journal of Family Psychotherapy,* 3, 73-91.

Schwebel, A.I. & Fine, M.A. (1994). *Understanding and helping families: A cognitive-behavioral approach.* Hillsdale, NJ: Lawrence Erlbaum Associates.

Infertility, "Experientially Oriented" Couples Therapy and Subsequent Pregnancy

Peggy J. Kleinplatz

SUMMARY. Four couples who had been diagnosed as clinically infertile were seen in experientially oriented couples therapy. Each couple conceived a baby shortly after a particularly powerful session. These sessions are described. The commonality across these sessions involved opening up the clients' inner experiencing and enabling these clients to actualize and integrate whatever was deeper within. The conventional biomedical and psychoanalytic approaches to infertility are described. The experiential model provides an alternative way to understand the timing of pregnancy or lack thereof. It also offers a holistic approach to working with infertile couples. *[Article copies available for a fee from The Haworth Document Delivery Service: 1-800-342-9678. E-mail address: getinfo@haworthpressinc.com <Website: http://www.haworthpressinc.com>]*

KEYWORDS. Infertility, conception, experiential model

Over the last year or so, I have been struck by the cases of four couples who conceived their children during the course of experientially oriented

Peggy J. Kleinplatz, PhD, teaches at the School of Psychology, University of Ottawa and at St. Paul University's Institute of Pastoral Studies. She has a private practice in sexual and couples therapy.

Address correspondence to: Peggy J. Kleinplatz, 161 Frank Street, Ottawa, Ontario K2P 0X4, Canada.

The author would like to thank Alvin R. Mahrer, PhD, for his constructive comments on earlier drafts of this article.

[Haworth co-indexing entry note]: "Infertility, 'Experientially Oriented' Couples Therapy and Subsequent Pregnancy." Kleinplatz, Peggy J. Co-published simultaneously in *Journal of Couples Therapy* (The Haworth Press, Inc.) Vol. 8, No. 2, 1999, pp. 17-35; and: *Couples and Pregnancy: Welcome, Unwelcome, and In-Between* (ed: Barbara Jo Brothers) The Haworth Press, Inc., 1999, pp. 17-35. Single or multiple copies of this article are available for a fee from The Haworth Document Delivery Service [1-800-342-9678, 9:00 a.m. - 5:00 p.m. (EST). E-mail address: getinfo@haworthpressinc.com].

couples therapy. Each conception occurred after a particularly powerful session that seemed to open some inner potential within one or both of the parents. What caught my attention was not only the timing of the pregnancies in relation to the therapy process but also that each of the couples had been diagnosed as clinically infertile.

Each couple had been in infertility treatment and none currently considered it likely that they would conceive. One woman had scarring of the fallopian tubes and adhesions throughout the pelvic cavity as a result of a severe case of pelvic inflammatory disease ten years earlier. Her husband had a vasectomy before he had met her, since reversed, but with a low sperm count and poor sperm motility. A second woman had both extensive external and internal scarring (i.e., covering her entire vulva, vagina, uterus, urinary tract, rectum, etc.) resulting from early, repeated and brutal childhood sexual abuse. A third had received surgical treatment for cervical cancer in her twenties and was now approaching forty. The fourth couple involved a husband with a low sperm count and a wife who had been unable to conceive either with her partner or through artificial insemination by donor.

I am hesitant about presenting these cases. I am not suggesting that the cause of infertility lies in psychopathology nor that psychotherapy provides a cure for infertility. Clearly, these four couples were ultimately able to conceive. I am also reluctant to fuel the blame and self-blame already heaped upon infertile couples (Gervaize, 1993; Mahlstedt, 1987). Yet perhaps there is more to conception or lack thereof and the timing of pregnancy than can be accounted for by biomedical approaches alone (Mahrer, 1978). Perhaps something deep within men, women or couples may be linked to the likelihood of conception. If we access and open it up in psychotherapy, one of the possible outcomes may include a greater chance of pregnancy.

PSYCHOLOGICAL ASPECTS OF INFERTILITY

Over the years, there has been a great deal of controversy surrounding the role of psychological factors in infertility. The tendency has been to understand the basis of infertility as either psychological or organic (cf. Seibel & Taymor, 1982). The therapist's theoretical orientation is closely related to how the therapist understands and works with issues surrounding pregnancy (Kleinplatz, 1992).

During the 1940s to 1960s, the literature in this area was dominated by psychoanalytic theory, attributing infertility to arrested female psychosexual development. There was no attention to male factors or to couples issues. In the 1960s up to 50% of infertility was explained as psychogenic (Eisner, 1963). More recently, the trend to interpret infertility as psychologically based has been reversed, with all or almost all infertility explained in biomedical terms (Domar, Seibel, Broome, Friedman & Zuttermeister, 1992; Domar & Seibel, 1990; Downey, 1993; Stewart & Robinson, 1989). The assumption that with advanced enough technology and diagnostic testing, all infertility will eventually be explained biomedically is ever-present (cf. Domar & Seibel, 1990; Harrison, O'Moore, O'Moore & McSweeney, 1981). Even the distress generated by infertility treatment and its possible role in the maintenance of infertility have been understood and described in biomedical (e.g., neuroendocrine) terms (Domar & Seibel, 1990; Domar, Seibel & Benson, 1990; Taymor, 1990).

Some warn of the harm that may result from insinuations that infertility may be psychogenic. Women could be pathologized out of a sexist bias as "hysterical, narcissistic and aggressive" (Greenfeld, Diamond, Breslin & DeCherney, 1987, p. 73). Others suggest caution in order to prevent infertile couples from feeling guilt, inadequacy and self-blame and to reduce the aspersions cast upon them by family and friends (Bell, 1983; Downey, 1993; Seibel & Taymor, 1982). Still others suggest exercising restraint in emphasizing psychological factors on scientific grounds (Takefman, 1990) or at least in order to be taken seriously by the scientific community (Taymor, 1990).

Most of the current literature dealing with psychological aspects of infertility focuses upon the impact of infertility and its treatment rather than the psychological factors contributing to infertility. Effects commonly listed include anxiety, stress, tension, hostility, grief, anger, frustration, depression, a sense of isolation, feeling out of control, guilt, decreased sexual self-esteem and self-efficacy, increased sexual dissatisfaction and dysfunction and marital distress (Andrews, Abbey & Halman, 1992; Black, Walther, Chute & Greenfeld, 1992; Boivin & Takefman, 1995; Boivin, Takefman, Tulandi & Brender, 1995; Burns, 1995; Domar & Seibel, 1990; Domar, Seibel et al., 1992; Greenfeld & Haseltine, 1986; Harrison, O'Moore et al., 1981; Koropatnick, Daniluk & Pattinson, 1993; McBain & Pepperell, 1987; Menning, 1980; Rosenthal, 1992; Seibel & Taymor, 1982; Stewart, Boydell, McCarthy, Swerdlyk, Redmond & Cohns, 1992). Treatment plans are generally intended to alleviate the above symptoms, particularly stress. The goal is to help individuals and couples adapt to and cope with treatment and/or the eventual loss of hope for conception. Programs typically involve educational and supportive counseling for individuals, couples and especially groups. The programs are oriented towards dealing with infertility, the treatment thereof and their effects (Andrews, Abbey et al., 1992; Bell, 1983; Downey, 1993; Rosenthal, 1992; Seibel & Taylor, 1982; Stewart, Boydell et al., 1992). Some include sexual therapy (Downey, 1993) or attention to grief work (Menning, 1980; Seibel & Taylor, 1982). One program incorporates relaxation training, stress management, cognitive restructuring, mindfulness (Domar, Seibel et al., 1990) with added peer support and a buddy system (Domar, Zuttermeister et al., 1992).

Although the majority of those working with infertile couples assume a biomedical position and recommend that the mental health professional help the couple adjust to their situation, a small contingent continues to explore the psychological origins and treatment of infertility (Cabau & Senarclens, 1986; Christie & Pawson, 1987, 1989; Pines, 1990a, 1990b, 1994; Sarrel & DeCherney, 1985; Taymor, 1990; Wasser, Sewall & Soules, 1993). Most of these are psychoanalytically oriented and tend to explain the basis of some infertility in terms of individual psychopathology. They cite such causal factors as repressed conflicts (Taymor, 1990), "mother fusion" and unrecognized fears of pregnancy (Sarrel & DeCherney, 1985), conflicts with father, hostility, phobic anxiety, psychosocial distress (Wasser, Sewall et al., 1993), unconscious ambivalence about their own mothers and about motherhood, and deep narcissistic wounds and psychosexual fixation (Pines, 1994). Infertility is seen as a "psychosomatic solution" to psychological conflict (Pines, 1990a).

A few are attuned to couples' psychodynamics as well as individual issues (Cabau & Senarclens, 1986; Christie and Pawson, 1987, 1989). Hidden and shared motivational conflicts may exist in individuals, between generations and within the couple. According to Christie and Pawson (1987, p. 327), "Infertility should always be seen as a conjugal phenomenon, i.e, one can justifiably speak of sterile marriages, rather than sterile individuals." Cabau & Senarclens (1986, p. 663) state, "Infertility can also be an integral part of the couple's relationship, and the unconscious refusal of pregnancy respects this."

For those who ascribe the origins of infertility to individual, couple or family dynamics, the suggested treatment is psychoanalytically oriented (Cabau & Senarclens, 1986; Christie & Pawson, 1987; Pines, 1990a, 1990b, 1994; Sarrel & DeCherney, 1985). The therapist's focus is on uncovering and interpreting the client's ambivalent relations with his/her own parents. To the extent that the infertility is psychogenic, it may be hazardous to treat the physiological symptom (i.e., the inability to conceive) by medical means. Such treatment may be ineffective and it will fail to treat the underlying problem (Pines, 1990b; Wasser, Sewall et al., 1993). Worse yet, if the treatment should "succeed" there are psychological risks to both the parents and the child who may subsequently be at risk for abuse (Christie & Pawson, 1989; Pines, 1994). "The dangers of an artificially induced pregnancy should not be under-estimated, as it can lead to breakdown through loss of defense mechanisms" (Cabau & Senarclens, 1986, p. 620).

In summary, there are two prevalent orientations in the literature to the causes and treatments of infertility. The major current approach explains the basis of infertility in biomedical terms. The recommended role for the therapist in this paradigm is to help clients adjust to the stressors of infertility, deal with the associated medical interventions and come to grips, if need be, with the permanence of their situation. The psychoanalytic perspective is currently a minority position, which holds that some infertility is psychogenic and suggests that therapists treat the underlying psychopathology.

THE EXPERIENTIAL MODEL

The approach I used with these four couples was experientially oriented couples therapy rather than either of the above paradigms. The experiential model does not explicitly discuss the origins of infertility nor does it aim to treat infertility. But its models of personality and human development (Mahrer, 1978) may provide a useful, alternative way of understanding conception or lack thereof. Experiential psychotherapy (Mahrer, 1983, 1986, 1996) may also offer therapists who work with infertile couples a holistic alternative to either of the two above approaches.

In the two prevalent orientations to infertility, one is working either with mind or body, treating either cause or effect. That is, in the biomedical approach, the primary problem is a biomedical disorder and the therapist aims to treat its psychological sequellae. From the psychoanalytic perspective, the therapist aims to treat the psychopathology which causes infertility. In contrast, in the experiential model, psychological states are neither the causes nor the effects of biomedical states. "Causality flows neither from bodily to behavioral, nor from behavioral to bodily; causality resides in [inner personality processes] which are expressed in *both* the behavioral and the bodily" (Mahrer, 1978, p. 157, emphasis in the original).

It is the client's inner experiencing or deeper potentials which govern the likelihood of conception. According to Mahrer, "Intercourse may result in conception, or it may not. Depending upon the person whom she is, depending on the way in which it is important for her world to be constructed, [the prospect of an infant] may be nurtured and developed, or it may wash away. . . . Her own potentials and their relationships determine whether an infant is to be constructed, or not" (Mahrer, 1978, p. 598). From this vantage point, conception, the timing of conception or lack thereof may be understood as expressions of potentials within the prospective parents as individuals or within the context of their relationship as a couple.

This approach attempts to promote the actualization and integration of the whole person. It does not aim to treat symptoms, problems or conditions (Mahrer, 1996). Rather it tries to achieve deep-seated change in the inner experiencing of the client. The two goals of each session are for the client to integrate the deeper potential, thereby becoming a "qualitatively new person" and for the client to be free of any painful feelings that were present at the start of the session (Mahrer, 1996, pp. 81-82). When these changes are accomplished, their ramifications may be evident in a myriad of ways, e.g., behaviourally, interpersonally and in the bodily state.

Thus, although the experiential approach does not set out to explain infertility, its models of personality and human development can allow us to speculate about the processes which may bring about or prevent conception. It is implicit that there would likely be individual differences in the particular processes or inner experiencing; these variations are to be regarded as just that, rather than as indications of psychopathology. Furthermore, paradoxically, although the experiential approach to psychotherapy does not endeavour to treat infertility, the nature of the changes it seeks are so profound and extensive that the results may just affect the client's subsequent chances of conception, (among other things). As such, this approach may be of interest to those who work with infertile couples.

WORKING WITH COUPLES IN EXPERIENTIAL PSYCHOTHERAPY

Experiential psychotherapy (Mahrer, 1986, 1993, 1996) was designed to be used with individuals, but it can be applied to couple and group therapy. Before describing these particular sessions, a brief description of experiential psychotherapy and how it may vary with couples may be in order.

In experiential psychotherapy, the therapist is aligned with the client and listens experientially. That is, the therapist is to be disengaged from her usual sense of self and allow the client's experiencing to flow through her. The first step in each session involves, "being in a moment of strong, full feelings and accessing or opening up an inner, deeper experiencing" (Mahrer & Roberge, 1993, p. 179). Once the inner experiencing has been welcomed and appreciated, the therapist's goal is to enable the client to become this deeper potential in the context of earlier life scenes (Mahrer, 1986). Finally, the patient is to, "have a taste of what it is like to be this whole new person, to think, act, feel and experience as this whole new person who is living and being in the world outside the office" (Mahrer, 1996, p. 337).

In using this approach with couples, the same general format is followed. However, it is the first and last step of each session which may sometimes differ from individual therapy. In working with couples, the moment of strong feelings may occur in the context of the interaction of the couple, during this session, when the feelings which begin to arise in one of them provide our initial focus. The compelling feelings emerging in either person in the course of the couple's interactions become our access and entry point to the inner experiencing. The therapist is attuned to pronounced feelings and begins to work intensively with which ever individual is beginning to show them. The middle of each session (i.e., welcoming and being the inner experiencing) are as described by Mahrer (1996). The presence of the partner tends to raise the stakes, heightening the intensity and allowing the observer a glimpse of the other's inner workings. There is something very special and risky about entering, exploring and expressing one's own depths while knowing that one's partner bears witness. It may serve to expand the intimacy in the relationship (Greenberg & Johnson, 1986, 1988; Schnarch, 1991). The concluding step involves having the client consider and try on for size the possibility of actually living as this new person, the inner experiencing, beyond this session. In this variation, the client also has the opportunity to include the partner and to experiment with or play out this new way of being with him/her, right then and there. Partners are typically receptive to these initiatives and tend to be eager to participate in the other's growth.

CASE ILLUSTRATIONS

Each of the couples conceived their child immediately after a particularly powerful therapy session (or in the case of Mr. and Mrs. Potter, after two such sessions, in which the first centered on Mr. Potter and the second centered on his wife).

Each of these five sessions will be described. The therapy processes and the changes that these clients underwent will then be discussed in terms of their possible relations to the subsequent pregnancies.

Ellen and John Potter

Mr. and Mrs. Potter had been referred to me by their family physician to deal with the impact of infertility and its treatment on their marital and sexual relations. During our first dozen sessions, we focused on their sexual difficulties, their destructive style of arguing, their meddling in-laws. It seems as though we have discussed everything but their feelings surrounding infertility. In our thirteenth session they enter arguing about the housework. She is saying, matter of factly, that he is irresponsible and that she always has to remind him to pull his share of the weight. As she continues, he withdraws, saying that he is apprehensive about fighting with her. He is afraid of her criticism and ridicule. (There are many options for the couples therapist at this point, including teaching fair fighting skills. In using this approach, given that Mr. Potter is beginning to show some feelings and they are growing, I choose to stay focused on them. At this point, the experiential work begins.) He describes the instants he hates most in fighting with his wife–the times when he just wants to bolt. He is feeling inadequate, useless, belittled and hurt, "like a little kid again." I am listening experientially, letting his words come through me and feeling myself shrink while another figure, nearby, is towering over me and berating me. I describe this aloud. "Yeah," he answers, "That's my father. It was always like that with him." I instruct him to talk to his father. As Mr. Potter attempts to do so, haltingly, my attention remains fixed on this big, cold, critical father. I ask, "What is he saying? What is he doing?" "He's not responding. He's running away," he answers with sorrow.

Mr. Potter chases after his father and confronts him, trying to get through to him. At the peak of a mostly one-sided dialogue with his father, what emerges is a sense of loving closeness and caring, touching and being touched. For Mr. Potter, this is the new, deeper experiencing. He remembers the rare occasions when he experienced these feelings in childhood. He is five years old and situated in a drab, musty garage. The smell of grease fills the air. He is watching intently as his father fixes the car. Mr. Potter is tinkering alongside his father as they chat leisurely about everything and nothing in particular. It is just the two of them and all that matters is being together. The moment seems precious and timeless. We search for and visit other such memories in his life, replete with this feeling and then return to the present and future. He contemplates calling his father and arranging for the two of them to leave their wives at home and go fishing together. "I love you, Dad and I want to have some happy times with you. I want to know about your life and your feelings. I want to be around when you're old and I want to take care of you. I want to show you that I love you before it's too late." He turns to his wife, saying that he wants to plan picnics with her and, one day, with any children they may have. "I cherish every minute I spend with you. I would die for you." He has long complained about job stressors but is now considering the possibility of switching positions in order to spend more time with his family. He is reaching out to his wife to hold him. He is beginning to cry. Mrs. Potter hugs him and says, "I love you."

He looks at her and asks, "Why do you love me? Will you love me no matter what I do?" She is crying now, too, and they are embracing one another.

"Just hug me more," he asks. Their voices are softening. She responds, "I love you so much. I can't imagine life without you."

He is gently stroking her face and hair, saying, "I have to have your touches every day . . . Every day. Even when you pat me on the bum it feels good . . . " Their words seems to be trailing off as they whisper in one another's ears and begin to kiss. The tenderness between them has grown intense enough for me to feel that I do not belong here. The moment is too intimate for my presence. I quietly leave my office as they continue to kiss and caress.

Their words have often suggested that they care about each other but rang hollow. He has typically treated her with resentment and animosity while she has generally regarded him with suspicion and self-righteousness. The inner feelings and corresponding behaviours which emerged in this session and in the following one are radical departures from their prior pattern of interactions.

In our next session, the subject turns to infertility. Mrs. Potter has just been invited to another baby shower, the fifth this year. She usually handles all the talk of maternity wear and nursery decor with grace but no more. "I'm tired of waiting," she says angrily. When her neighbour, Martha, announced another pregnancy, Mrs. Potter froze. "I didn't want to be polite. It's not fair. I just know we'd make such good parents." Listening experientially, (i.e., letting Mrs. Potter's words come through me and allowing them to evoke images, feelings and sensations) my gaze is fixed on Martha's belly. The feelings are of loss, emptiness, being incomplete; something is missing. She is crying softly. "It's just not fair. There are all these parents who ship their kids off to day care every day. John and I would never do that and yet we can't have a baby." As she continues to describe the kind of parent that she will never be, I am allowing her words to flow through me. Her words transport me to being a brand new mother. I am suffused with the possibility of being captivated by a precious little one, of being different from all those people who take their kids for granted, of cherishing my special child. I describe aloud the joy of holding this newborn baby, being enraptured by her, counting her fingers and toes, unable to look away. She hesitates, asking why she should talk about motherhood when it seems impossible. I respond that the choice is hers alone, but that these powerful, magical feelings are right there, within reach. I invite her to allow herself, for just a moment, to feel all the love she has on hold. I return to describing being absolutely overwhelmed by how special this child is, of carrying the whole world of possibilities in my arms.

Mrs. Potter responds that she recognizes these feelings but experiences them rarely. "The last time was two years ago, just before Christmas. My brother and his family were staying with us. I was baking cookies when Evan, the four-year old, asked if he could help. He was trying to crack some eggs and I was holding his hand and showing him how you do it, really patiently. He tried to do one by himself and he ended up with yolk all over his little fingers and egg shells everywhere. He looked up at me and I had this incredible feeling come over me and I said to him that I love him." We enter into this memory, making it alive and vivid. We linger long enough to feel the warm glow of cherishing this small child, who still has egg yolk dripping from his gooey fingers. He seems a little baffled by the outpouring of affection but that only makes him seem more adorable.

Soon after, I encourage her to search for other, similar moments, wherein she felt overwhelmed by a sense of fascination, appreciation and loving warmth. She recalls and enters into a series of such memories, mostly from childhood, involving other people but also her cats.

After the marvelling adoration has peaked, I address this seemingly new woman, the one immersed in combing the thick, grey fur of the cat nestled in her lap. I ask her to imagine how different it might be if only *she* could take charge of Mrs. Potter's life. She responds, "I would be more loving, more affectionate, physically and verbally, with my family. I really value my brother, but I rarely show it. Maybe I could hug him when I see him. He's usually so stiff but I could do it, even if he gets all flustered. And I could throw my arms around John when he gets home from work. I'm usually complaining about my day when he walks in but instead, I could tell him how much he means to me every chance I get."

I add, "Why wait till 5:00 PM? What about calling him at work and saying, "I want you . . ."" "Now. At home," she interjects. She is speaking adoringly with just a shade of seductiveness. There is an immediacy bordering on urgency in her tone. The love is overflowing. She turns to John. She has gone beyond merely contemplating how she could be in the future; she is ready to share these feelings with John right now. "I could watch you sleep. I could watch you while you're sleeping and stroke your shoulders. And when you open your eyes," she says, with tears welling up, "I'd be lying there next to you, loving you."

Mrs. Potter considers how to deal with the next announcement of a neighbour's pregnancy. "I'm going to call John and make baby talk with him." She is looking at him intently and cooing to him as if he were a small child. She reaches over to touch him tenderly.

He begins to respond, saying, "I feel so close to you. You're a special person. I just feel lucky." They are gazing into one another's eyes. The rest of the world, including me, has receded into non-existence. They are holding each other and crying quietly.

Mike and Nancy Kelly

Ms. Kelly had been physically and sexually abused from earliest childhood through adolescence. The incest had been brutal enough to leave extensive scarring and a diagnosis of infertility. She and her husband are attempting to deal with the long-term impact of the abuse on their marriage in terms of the infertility and their sex life. They love one another deeply but their sexual relations are infrequent, physically painful, emotionally distant and unfulfilling. Ms. Kelly had been able to engage in arousing, exciting sex with total strangers in the past or as she worded it, "There was something inside of me that would do these bad things." She sees sex with someone she loves as a contradiction in terms. "It was easier before getting married. Now I space out. I'm numb. Mike deserves better than that."

In this session she begins with the recurrent pain she feels in her vagina and rectum. The images dominating the early part of the session involve being locked in the basement by her uncle. She is screaming as he rapes and beats her. She is approximately three years old. The feelings are of being invaded, tortured, contaminated and damaged. As I allow her words to come through me, I am being coldly vivisected. Things are stuck inside. As the sharp, stabbing pain increases, she moves into a different sets of feelings: Being painfully empty, detached, "unreal," "dizzy," "a zombie." "When I disappear my eyes are only half open. I don't want to see too much." (This is how she endures having sex with her husband.)

As we alternate between the initial torment and the inaccessible numbness, a new, deeper set of feelings emerges. It involves a sense of spaciousness and "opening up," of soaring expansiveness and weightlessness. At one instant we are swimming under water, gliding and submerging effortlessly. In the next we are floating and seeing stars. There are no limits. "You can do it anywhere." And indeed, she recalls being confined and abused in the basement by day and chasing the stars in the sky by night as she lay by the bedroom window in childhood. By the end of the session the pain has disappeared and is replaced by the sense of being on the verge of total freedom and expansiveness. The surge of energy and intense vitality provide stark contrast to the former deadness. She imagines, "living more, instead of just surviving and working on incest . . . and finally making space for our life together."

At the next session, both sets of feelings that dominated previously are gone, as is the accompanying physical pain. Instead, Mr. and Ms. Kelly are now making contact during sex. "It feels risky but not scary." Furthermore, the dyspareunia is gone. "Sexually, I'm more in my body and I am present with Mike. I can look at him and let him inside me. It's really something to find that someone who knows me as well as Mike would still want me . . . There is more room for others now. The circle is getting a bit larger." Shortly thereafter, Mr. and Ms. Kelly announce that they are expecting a baby.

Gerald and Karen Williams

Both Mr. and Mrs. Williams were brought up in homes dominated by physical and sexual abuse, although only the daughters were sexually abused in each family. They have had long-standing difficulties with intimacy and sexuality, aggravated in recent years by infertility.

In our fourth session, Mr. Williams begins with the old, familiar feelings of being an outsider in the home, of being misunderstood, frustrated and alone within his family. He recalls being seven years old and standing in the kitchen as his step-father approaches menacingly. He is feeling threatened, cornered and intimidated. We flesh out this memory, making it vivid and fresh, searching for its emotional peak. His step-father teases and goads him and he begins to squirm in shame. As his step-father continues to needle him, he is feeling increasingly demeaned, bizarre, a reject, a "twisted pervert." He has remembered such moments countless times. But now, living in this moment, something new emerges in this memory. It is when he looks at his mother, sitting silently and pathetically in the background, that he imagines how it might have felt to turn to her and to reach out to her with warmth and affection. He speaks with her now, saying the words he never spoke aloud in childhood. He asks her to leave his step-father so that they might have a chance of belonging together. As we enter into this dialogue with his mother, new feelings of loving intimacy and connection arise and grow more pronounced. At first there is sadness, accompanied by tears, for missed opportunities–what might have been. But he soon remembers sharing these kinds of moments with his grandfather, his gym teacher and others in childhood. The man whose relationships have been dominated by alienation and isolation is gone. He becomes the boy who reaches out and takes the initiative to connect with those he loves. "I've had little tidbits of these euphoric feelings in my life but where are they now? I have the capacity for love and affection, honesty and intimacy that I haven't even tapped into!"

He begins to picture the future and is filled with eager anticipation at the possibilities ahead. We start with mere sketches but fill them in with enough detail and colour to make them excitingly viable. He imagines reaching out to his older sister, various friends and colleagues and expressing the fondness and desire to be close with them that is usually muted. He envisions visiting his grandfather's grave, overflowing with love and talking to him, telling him how much he appreciated his grandfather's caring and how he became an architect to be just like him. He kneels by the gravestone, carefully placing a handful of daisies nearby. He considers confronting his family about the anger he still harbours alongside the love he longs to share.

At the outset of our next session, he reports that he has followed through on all the possibilities he had considered. Furthermore, he suddenly found others reciprocating. "Is it synchronicity? Am I sending out messages that others are picking up?" He had gone further than originally planned, allowing himself to feel and express sexual desire with Karen. "I just let myself be myself around her . . . I reached out to her and she responded to me . . . I felt so centered. I felt so clear." Two weeks later, he and his wife announce that they are expecting a baby.

Anne and Jason Davis

Mr. and Mrs. Davis have always wanted children. That is why they married one another, though each has been reluctant to acknowledge this. They speak of being guarded with one another and of the walls between them. Mr. Davis reached middle age without marrying or ever leaving his mother's home. Mrs. Davis has been through a series of disastrous relationships. In her last marriage, she had been step-mother to a girl, Ellen, whom she had raised almost single-handedly for three years, until the age of four. But when she and her ex-husband divorced, he retained sole custody of his daughter and left the province. She married Mr. Davis in the hope of having a baby as soon as possible. She has never dealt with the loss of Ellen nor with the impact of the subsequent diagnosis and treatment for infertility. "It's just too painful."

Her life is a series of battlegrounds, with "useless," "incompetent," "irritants" surrounding her. These include her employees, the dog and her husband. He complains that she belittles and demeans him: "She treats me like a child."

"You *are* a bit of a mummy's boy," she responds in exasperation. She is condescending and insulting, taunting him to grow up.

In this, our second session, her feelings are of being stressed, of spinning her wheels, of running but not getting anywhere. All around there is noise that never lets up. When she focuses on the constant stream of motion, she becomes aware of a sense of being inert, of silence and loneliness. She feels heavy, insulated and protected. (She has gained 25 lb. in the last year.) As the feeling intensifies, it seems harder to breathe, almost stifling. I encourage her to let it overwhelm her and to describe whatever images may arise in the course of these feelings and sensations. She responds with images of her former step-daughter. "I'm carrying this weight to protect myself from loss of Ellen." I begin searching aloud for Ellen, wanting to see her again. Mrs. Davis is looking at Ellen wistfully, with a sweet longing, a yearning for this child and their relationship. "She was at such a perfect stage . . . Out of diapers but still cuddly and wanting to hold my hand in public." Mrs. Davis is letting herself miss Ellen, allowing herself to be content in wishing for more. She is reaching out, extending herself, going beyond herself and moving towards children, wanting to connect and be close with children. "It's children that make you loving." Although she had dreaded even thinking about Ellen, the feelings are now soft, full, easy, flowing and peaceful. She is welcoming and immersing herself in them. The inclination to race about is gone as is the sense of being heavy and stifled.

Mrs. Davis returns to the present and looks at her husband curiously. She is shifting away from venturing forward and seeking closeness–such feelings do not fit for her in relation to Mr. Davis–but then her usual impatience and aggravation with him is absent, too. She is seeing him afresh and differently. "It's not you. The issue is Ellen and everything else is coming from that. In the meantime, I don't have an awful lot of love to give you, Jason. I haven't been very gracious . . . I want to be with you and treat you with respect." He seems touched and relieved, saying that he loves her and is willing to wait for more.

In the session that follows, Mr. and Mrs. Davis report that the sexual attraction for one another and mutual respect are growing. Soon after, they announce the pregnancy.

DISCUSSION

I was surprised and delighted when these four couples announced their pregnancies. I had not been attempting to treat infertility, nor was I offering a program for couples to deal with the stressors caused by infertility. My only "plan" was to start with whatever feelings emerged in the early part of each session and to allow these to determine the focus and directions for change for the duration of that session. I did not anticipate or aim for conception. How are these pregnancies and the timing of them to be understood? What happened in these sessions that may help to account for these pregnancies? What are the implications for working with infertile couples in therapy?

In trying to understand the factors that may have contributed to these pregnancies, I searched for commonalities among these clients across all five sessions. The focus at the outset of each session varied, as did the initial feelings. There was no predominant emphasis on infertility across the opening, middle or end points of the sessions. The inner experiencing in four of the five sessions could be described, loosely, as involving vaguely, similar feelings of intimacy and love. However, there are certainly differences between moments of timeless togetherness and sharing versus being captivated, enraptured, with adoring fascination and as compared with wistful yearning, longing and reaching out.

What seems to characterize all of these sessions is the process that the clients underwent. The initial focus of each session was determined by what was front and center for the particular clients at the time. I attended to whatever was stirring in my clients and allowed that to direct us within. This differs from the literature which recommends that the therapist structure treatment around relaxation training, coping strategies, grief work, educational counselling, etc. The second and major commonality among these sessions is that we searched for whatever was deeper within the clients; each client was enabled to become this inner experiencing and to incorporate this new way of being in his/her relationships outside the therapy office. Although the specific nature of the inner experiencing varied among the clients, each person opened up some deeper potential and entered into being it fully and with intense, good feelings. By the end, the clients were free of the emotional and/or physical pain that dominated at the outset and were able to envision new ways of being in the future.

The profound changes these clients went through affected several different areas of their lives. For these individuals, the changes included modifying career plans, devoting more time to family and friends, elimination of bodily pain and increased sexual desire. For these couples, the changes involved more openness and honesty and qualitative improvements in sexual and intimate contact. Those who witnessed their partners' experiential work seemed to acquire greater understanding of their partners. They appeared to be touched by their partners' explorations, appreciative of their courage and responsive to opportunities to share in their growth.

When clients become their inner experiencings, the depth and breadth of their changes may be quite extensive. When these changes are sufficiently significant and powerful, they may transform aspects of clients' lives (Mahrer, 1993, 1996). Changes and their ramifications may be manifest in unexpected ways, some of which may never have been discussed or considered explicitly in therapy. These cases raise the possibility that perhaps one of the consequences of such deep-seated change may be a readiness for pregnancy and conception. When clients undergo full actualization and integration of what had previously been out of reach within, when it becomes a welcome part of their daily experiencing, its prior bodily expresssion may evaporate (Mahrer, 1978, p. 171). Furthermore, the change(s) may occur in the wife or, in contrast with the traditional psychoanalytic view, in the husband and/or in the couple.

There are, no doubt, other possible ways of describing, explaining or dismissing these four, unexpected pregnancies. There are several advantages to using the experiential model as a way of understanding these events, for those so inclined (i.e., for those who have concerns about the limitations and implications of either the biomedical or psychoanalytic orientations). Firstly, clients who have been diagnosed as infertile need not be pathologized. They need not be seen as suffering from either mechanical failure or serious psychological problems. We can go beyond biomedical perspectives on infertility without resorting to notions of psychopathology. Secondly, the persons who want children can be understood and approached holistically rather than being reduced to minds versus bodies or bodily parts. The experiential model provides an alternative to dualistic "either-or" outlooks. The timing of pregnancy may be seen in terms of mind and body working together to express the inner experiencing. Thirdly, fertility/infertility may reflect the deeper potentials of either partner or both of them in combination. Attributions of infertility and the focus of treatment need not center on the prospective mother.

For psychotherapists, one of the implications of these cases may be that when working with infertile couples, consider trying experientially oriented couples therapy in addition to or instead of the existing approaches. That is, instead of treating the psychological symptoms caused by the stress of infertility, helping couples adapt to their situation or treating the underlying psychopathology that may be causing the infertility, consider the experiential alternative. This entails offering therapy to whole persons and aiming for growth based on whatever is on their minds and is deeper within. Rather than treating causes versus effects, we can reach for transformation. Regardless of whether or not the focus of the session seems to be infertility, when the changes are impressively deep-seated and extensive, one of the possible results may include subsequent pregnancy.

SUMMARY AND CONCLUSIONS

Four clinically infertile couples were seen in experientially oriented couples therapy. Each couple unexpectedly conceived just after a particularly powerful session. Although there were no obvious commonalities in the content of subject matter among these sessions, a pattern is apparent when examining the therapy process. Each client focused upon what was front and center for him/her at the beginning of the session. In each session the clients accessed and became their inner experiencing fully and intensely. They became free of the painful feelings that had troubled them at the outset and seemed qualitatively different. They were then able to envision integrating these new ways of being beyond therapy. The important and extensive changes occurring in these individuals and couples may have contributed towards the subsequent conceptions.

Therapists may wish to consider replacing or adding to the conventional treatments for infertile couples. The experiential model provides a holistic alternative to the current approaches to the understanding and treatment of infertility. Therapists may want to be open to focusing on and delving into whatever is going on within their clients, rather than structuring treatment around stress management, coping techniques or stages of mourning. This approach goes beyond treating causes, symptoms or effects of either psychological or biomedical disorders; it opens the door to changes in behaviour, relationships and in the body that could never have been anticipated from treating only the presenting problem. When clients are enabled to become whatever is deeper, the profound changes may transform the lives of the individuals, the couple and may just enable them to conceive.

REFERENCES

Andrews, F.M., Abbey, A., & Halman, L.J. (1992). Is fertility-problem stress different? The dynamics of stress in fertile and infertile couples. *Fertility and Sterility*, 57(6), 1247-1253.

Bell, J.S. (1983). Psychological aspects. In T.B. Hargreave (Ed.), *Male Infertility*, (pp. 46-55). New York: Springer-Verlag.

Black, R.B., Walther, V.N., Chute, D. & Greenfeld, D.A. (1992). When in vitro fertilization fails: A prospective view. *Social Work in Health Care, 17*(3), 1-19.

Boivin, J. & Takefman, J.E. (1995). Stress level across stages of in vitro fertilization in subsequently pregnant and nonpregnant women. *Fertility and Sterility, 64* (4), 802-810.

Boivin, J., Takefman, J.E., Tulandi, T. & Brender, W. (1993). Reactions to infertility based on extent of treatment failure. *Fertility and Sterility. 63*(4), 801-807.

Burns, L.H. (1995). An overview of the sexual dysfunction in the infertile couple. *Journal of Family Psychotherapy, 6*(1), 25-46.

Cabau, A. & Senarclens, M. de (1986). Psychological aspects of infertility. In V. Insler & B. Lunenfeld (Eds.), *Infertility: Male and female* (pp. 648-673). New York: Churchill Livingstone.

Christie, G.L. & Pawson, M.E. (1987). The psychological and social management of the infertile couple. In R.J. Pepperell, B. Hudson & C. Wood (Eds.), *The infertile couple* (pp. 313-339). New York: Churchill Livingstone.

Christie, G.L. & Pawson, M. (1989). Barren womanhood: Psychological aspects of infertility. In P. Ashurst & Z. Hall (Eds.), *Understanding women in distress* (pp. 104-114). New York: Routledge.

Domar, A.D. & Seibel, M.M. (1990). Emotional aspects of infertility. In M.M. Seibel (Ed.), *Infertility: A comprehensive text* (pp. 23-35). Norwalk, Connecticut: Appleton & Lange.

Domar, A.D., Seibel, M.M. & Benson, H. (1990). The mind/body program for infertility: A new behavioral treatment approach for women with infertility. *Fertility and Sterility, 53*(2), 246-249.

Domar, A.D., Seibel, M., Broome, A., Friedman, R. & Zuttermeister, P.C. (1992). The prevalence and predictability of depression in infertile women. *Fertility and Sterility, 58* (6), 1158-1163.

Domar, A.D., Zuttermeiseter, P.C., Seibel, M. & Benson, H. (1992). Psychological improvement in infertile women after behavioral treatment: A replication. *Fertility and Sterility, 58* (1), 144-147.

Downey, J. (1993). Infertility and the new reproductive technologies. In D.E. Stewart & N.L. Stotland (Eds.), *Psychological aspects of women's health care: The interface between psychiatry and obstetrics and gynecology* (pp. 193-206). Washington, D.C.: American Psychiatric Press.

Eisner, B.G. (1963). Some psychological differences between fertile and infertile women. *Journal of Clinical Psychology, 19, 391.*

Gervaize, P.A. (1993). The psychosexual impact of fertility and its treatment. *Canadian Journal of Human Sexuality, 2* (3), 141-147.

Greenberg, L.S. & Johnson, S.M. (1986). Emotionally focused couples therapy. In N.S. Jacobson & A.S. Gurman (Eds.), *Clinical handbook of marital therapy* (pp. 253-276). New York: Guilford.

Greenberg, L.S. & Johnson, S.M. (1988). *Emotionally focused therapy for couples.* New York: Guilford.

Greenfeld, D., Diamond, M.P., Breslin, R.L. & DeCherney, A. (1986). Infertility and the new reproductive technology: A role for social work. *Social Work in Health Care, 12* (2), 71-81.

Greenfeld, D. & Haseltine, F. (1986). Candidate selection and psychosocial considerations of in-vitro fertilization procedures. *Clinical Obstetrics and Gynecology, 29* (1), 119-126.

Harrison, R.F., O'Moore, A.M., O'Moore, R.R. & McSweeney, J.R. (1981). Stress profiles in normal infertile couples: Pharmacological and psychological approaches to therapy (pp. 143-157). In V. Insler & G. Bettendorf (Eds.), *Advances in diagnosis and treatment of infertility.* New York: Elsevier/North-Holland.

Kleinplatz, P.J. (1992). The pregnant clinical psychologist: Issues, impressions and observations. *Women and Therapy, 12* (1/2), 21-37.

Koropatnick, S., Daniluk, J. & Pattinson, H.A. (1993). Infertility: A non-event transition. *Fertility and Sterility, 59* (1), 163-171.

Mahlstedt, P.P. (1987). The crisis of infertility: An opportunity for growth. In G. Weeks & L. Hof (Eds.), *Integrating sex and marital therapy* (pp. 121-148). New York: Brunner/Mazel.

Mahrer, A.R. (1978). *Experiencing: A humanistic theory of psychology and psychiatry.* New York: Brunner/Mazel.

Mahrer, A.R. (1986). *Therapeutic experiencing: The process of change.* New York: Norton.

Mahrer, A .R. (1993). Transformational psychotherapy sessions. *Journal of Humanistic Psychology, 33* (2), 30-37.

Mahrer, A.R. (1996). *The complete guide to experiential psychotherapy.* New York: Wiley.

Mahrer, A.R. & Roberge, M. (1993). Single-session experiential therapy with any person whatsoever. In R.A. Wells & V.J. Gionetti (Eds.), *Casebook of the brief therapies* (pp. 179-196). New York: Plenum.

McBain, J.C. & Pepperell, R.J. (1987). Unexplained infertility. In R.J. Pepperell, B. Hudson & C. Wood (Eds.), *The Infertile Couple* (pp. 208-221). New York: Churchill Livingstone.

Menning, B.E. (1980). The emotional needs of infertile couples. *Fertility and Sterility, 34* (4), 313-319.

Pines, D. (1990a). Pregnancy, miscarriage and abortion: A psychoanalytic perspective. *International Journal of Psychoanalysis, 71,* 301-307.

Pines, D. (1990b). Emotional aspects of infertility and its treatment. *International Journal of Psychoanalysis, 71,* 561-568.

Pines, D. (1994). *A woman's unconscious use of her body.* New Haven: Yale University Press.

Robinson, G.E. & Stewart, D.E. (1989). Motivation for motherhood and the experience of pregnancy. *Canadian Journal of Psychiatry, 34,* 861-865.

Rosenthal, M.B. Infertility: Psychotherapeutic issues. *New Directions for Mental Health Services, 55,* 61-71.

Sarrel, P.M. & DeCherney, A.H. (1985). Psychotherapeutic intervention for treatment of couples with secondary infertility. *Fertility and Sterility, 43,* (6), 897-900.

Schnarch, D. (1991). *Constructing the sexual crucible: An integration of sexual and marital therapy.* New York: Norton.

Seibel, M.M. & Taymor, M. (1982). Emotional aspects of infertility. *Fertility and Sterility, 37* (2), 137-145.

Shapiro, C.H. (1988). *Infertility and pregnancy loss*. San Francisco: Jossey-Bass.

Stewart, D.E., Boydell, K.M., McCarthy, K., Swerdlyk, S., Redmond, C. & Cohrs, W. (1992). A prospective study of the effectiveness of brief professionally-led support groups for infertility patients. *International Journal of Psychiatry in Medecine, 22* (2), 173-182.

Stewart, D.E. & Robinson, G.E. (1989). Infertility by choice or by nature. *Canadian Journal of Psychiatry, 34*, 866-871.

Takefman, J. (1990). Behavioral treatment for infertile women: Letter to the editor. *Fertility and Sterility, 54* (6), 1183.

Taymor, M.L. (1990). *Infertility: A clinician's guide to diagnosis and treatment*. New York: Plenum.

Wasser, S.K., Sewall, G. & Soules, M.R. (1993). Psychosocial stress as a cause of infertility. *Fertility and Sterility, 59* (3), 685-689.

Catastrophic Conditions in Couple Systems: Managing an Unwelcome Pregnancy

Barbara J. Lynch

SUMMARY. A presentation of case studies forms the focus for an exploration of the discovery of an abortion or adoption used as the management of an unwelcome pregnancy which occurred in the context of the marital system. Managing an impasse in the middle phase of therapy in each case led to the emergence of information which then allowed the therapist to work with the couple system to alleviate the core situation out of which presenting problems emanated. In these cases the unwelcome pregnancy had the potential to be cataclysmic to the couple system. Therefore, the possibility that a couple is concealing an abortion or an adoption should be considered by couples' therapists when there is little or no response to usual strategies for change. The reason for concealment is immaterial. What is paramount is that the therapist bring the event to the fore of treatment and work with a couple to put closure on what is generally an unresolved issue. *[Article copies available for a fee from The Haworth Document Delivery Service: 1-800-342-9678. E-mail address: getinfo@haworthpressinc.com <Website: http://www.haworthpressinc.com>]*

KEYWORDS. Pregnancy, adoption, abortion, grief

INTRODUCTION

The marital system, in a manner similar to other systems, is prone to disruptions of varying degrees of severity which have a range of effects from

Barbara J. Lynch is Professor, Southern Connecticut State University, Department of Marriage and Family Therapy, 501 Crescent Street, New Haven, CT 06515.

[Haworth co-indexing entry note]: "Catastrophic Conditions in Couple Systems: Managing an Unwelcome Pregnancy." Lynch, Barbara J. Co-published simultaneously in *Journal of Couples Therapy* (The Haworth Press, Inc.) Vol. 8, No. 2, 1999, pp. 37-48; and: *Couples and Pregnancy: Welcome, Unwelcome, and In-Between* (ed: Barbara Jo Brothers) The Haworth Press, Inc., 1999, pp. 37-48. Single or multiple copies of this article are available for a fee from The Haworth Document Delivery Service [1-800-342-9678, 9:00 a.m. - 5:00 p.m. (EST). E-mail address: getinfo@haworthpressinc.com].

low level disturbances to fatal catastrophes. The basic foundation of an intimate system is a deciding factor in determining the degree of devastation present after the trigger event has abated. There are some situations which have consequences no matter how innately healthy the system may be. These occurrences inevitably have a destructive impact of the marital system and frequently the relationship does not survive.

Conditions that portent relationship destruction could be those that come along by means of inherited predispositions. This includes tendencies toward structuring the relationship according to hierarchical inequities; a learned unwillingness to make emotional expression a part of intimate relating; rigid gender role expectations, and numerous others. Systems with these characteristics usually erode over time, taking several years to reach a state of complete dissipation. The manifest characteristics are insidious. The basic foundation of the relationship slowly disintegrates until, seemingly suddenly, the entire structure collapses. The presenting problems that emerge from these systems prior to an extreme exacerbation, respond extremely well to either preventative measures, relationship enhancement endeavors, or to marital therapy.

Many fairly healthy couples often seek intervention before the onset of major symptoms. However, many couples are not motivated to initiate the steps necessary to insure an avoidance of serious relationship ruin until some loss has already been experienced. These couples come to therapy nearly too late, ready to defeat a therapist's best effort.

Other conditions, more destructive to the couple system, emerge as a response to outside forces. While the basic soundness of the relationship continues to have a part in determining the degree of destruction, there are usually no effective preventative measures against a severe response. Random victimization, rape, the death of a child all can be classified as ravagers of a relationship. These events have the power to consume many areas of intimacy, leaving either a hollow shell of a relationship or an irrevocable severing of all emotional ties. However, even in the aftermath of these catastrophic events, a sound marital system can response positively to well timed, effective therapy.

There are also those conditions which combine pre-existing relationship factors with those outside the boundaries of the couple system. An extra-marital affair carries with it a betrayal of trust and a disintegration of individual and system worth. The degree of damage sustained by the marital system is not predetermined. There will be an impact; however, the affair can be either an initiator of change in the relationship or the means to end the marriage. Many factors enter into which outcome occurs and therapy can play a significant role in the potential result.

The management of an unwelcome pregnancy occurring within the boundaries of the system, not the result of an outside liaison, is a factor which has definite consequences of varying degrees of severity affected by several variables. Foremost among these variables is the choice to either make the resulting infant a part of the system or to intentionally exclude the child either by abortion or adoption. The process by which this decision is made within the couple system and the ongoing impact of this decision alter the compexion of intimacy in all cases.

Therapists are well aware of the potential for difficulty that an unwelcome pregnancy presents to a couple system. When a couple is not forthcoming with this information, and the therapist does not specifically inquire about unwelcome pregnancies, a full understanding of the context of the presenting problem remains unavailable. Without being able to locate the presenting problem, a therapist may explore several areas of relationship dysfunction and still be left with a dissatisfied couple and no appreciable change in their system.

Following a series of fruitless interventions or minor "cosmetic" changes that do not significantly alleviate the basic marital discontent, both couple and therapist tend to be frustrated. The couple has the option of leaving treatment and seeking out another therapist or type of therapy. The therapist must manage the treatment failure in any one of several ways, some more functional that others.

The sole premise of this paper is to heighten the therapist's awareness of a possible avenue to explore when reasonable attempts to move past a therapeutic impasse have failed. Three case studies are presented to alert the therapist to the therapeutic possibilities that emerge as a result of inquiring about and exploring the circumstances around an unwelcome pregnancy within the couple system. There is no specific new intervention strategy to employ in treatment. Most psychiatric nurses and nurse practitioners doing psychotherapy routinely elicit information about pregnancies and follow up with specific questions about miscarriages, abortions, stillbirths, etc. This is different from most psychotherapists who request the number of children in a family and may follow up with more direct questions about a variety of related topics. However, it is not routine for most marriage and family therapists to request information about the presence and management of unwelcome pregnancies that occurred within the context of the marriage under treatment. Without regard for the morality, legality, or the ethics of abortion or adoption, this is vital relationship information that is germane to treatment. The therapist is inquiring about a catastrophic couple event, one which attacks the relationship with tremendous force. The following three case studies will illustrate this.

PREMARITAL PREGNANCY AND THE ADOPTION CHOICE

Carol and Bruce were high school seniors whose relationship had intensified to the point where they were considering becoming engaged upon graduation and being married sometime during their college years. Once this decision had been made, sex became an accepted part of their intimacy. Shortly before graduation, Carol discovered that she was pregnant. The couple wasn't upset about this development. Rather they viewed it as a catalyst to beginning their future as a couple sooner than they had anticipated. Neither of them factored in the reactions of their families when they separately told them about the pregnancy. Both Carol and Bruce had been counting on their parent's emotional and financial support as vital to the success of their future and that of their expected child. They could not have been more shocked by the outcome of conversing with their parents. Both sets of parents were vehemently opposed to their children's plans. Not only were they unwilling to be forthcoming with any form of support, they actively militated an end to all aspects of the relationship; the intimacy, the pregnancy, and the plans for marriage. Bruce's parents immediately made their position clear and backed it up with action. They gave Bruce a choice. If he did not give up this relationship with Carol, he would not get any financial backing for college and furthermore he would be completely banished from the family. He was an only child of aging parents and this combination of threats required more strength and more maturity than he possessed to defy. He was incapable of functioning without their support. Carol's father simply cowered her with physical and emotional abuse to the point where she was banished to her room, forbidden to have any contact with Bruce or anyone outside her family. Within three months of the announcement, Bruce's father sought out to corporate transfer which allowed the family to move two thousand miles away in an attempt to insure that the young could/would have no contact.

Through the clandestine efforts of Carol's younger sister, the couple communicated briefly by letter. Bruce swore undying love for Carol, telling her that he would get back to her at his first opportunity when he was able to be fully supportive of her. He promised her that they would have children in the future to take the place of this one that was being taken from them. Carol reciprocated his love and promised to wait for him. The interactive portion of the couple's relationship ended.

Carol was sequestered during most of her pregnancy. Her family's strong Catholic beliefs offered no choice except to deliver the child and place it for adoption. She was maintained on house "arrest" with another family member on guard to be sure she made no contact with outsiders. When her delivery date was close, her father accompanied her to a relative in a distant state where he deposited her to give birth and to follow through on adoption plans. Following long and arduous labor, she gave birth to a healthy daughter whom she held briefly and then turned over to a social worker, beginning the process of legally severing all ties to the infant. Two weeks later she returned home to begin a four year life of quiet depression.

True to his word, Bruce completed college with an engineering degree and again, with the help of Carol's younger sister, got word to her that they were now able to resume their aborted plans for a future together. Carol's family had relaxed their vigilance of her activity since they had come to view her as a repentant sinner who had learned the error of her ways and was now compliant to the family wishes. This allowed her to simply walk out, meet Bruce in another city and eventually have a civil marriage ceremony. Both families, once recovered form their initial distress, were so impressed by the tenacious way the couple kept their commitment to each other, that they rescinded their disapproval and welcomed the couple to the family. They eventually went so far as insisting that the couple have a religious ceremony to publicly begin their marriage. The daughter and granddaughter all three families had given up was never mentioned. It was as if it had never happened.

A son was born to Carol and Bruce after they had been married for six years and had almost given up hope that they would become parents ever again. Although they never mentioned the previous time they had conceived a child, it was present in metaphor, and rarely far from their thoughts. It was as if they remembered to forget. It wasn't until the birth of their second child was imminent, when their son was five years old, that the past contaminated the present. Carol became almost possessed with an irrational fear that the marriage would end along with some strange, unexpressed, wish that it would. Eventually the situation became unbearable and the couple sought out therapy.

After several unproductive sessions, when the therapist finally professed to be at a loss to initiate some meaningful change, Carol spewed out her story. She confessed to being desperately afraid that the daughter she had given up for adoption would come searching for her birth parents and she wanted to have this unknown child find her parents intact in an admirable relationship. At the same time she realized that her abandoned daughter was the same age that she herself had been at the time of her conception and Carol had the illogical idea that he daughter might get pregnant and repeat the pattern. She believed she needed to warn her. Finally, the expected baby was due close to the birthday of her first child, the lost daughter. Carol had a need for this baby to replace the daughter she abandoned and was convinced that the child was a female even though she had refused to be told the gender when the knowledge was available to her via her ultra-sound examination. In the midst of all the intrusion from the past onto the present, Carol confessed that she really hadn't forgiven Bruce for abandoning her and their baby and she wasn't sure if she could ever love him again. The baby was born before another session could be scheduled and it was a boy. At the next session Carol announced that she was going to initiate divorce proceedings. There was no hope of saving their marriage. A three year bitter legal battle ensued during which Carol decided to give up custody of her sons to Bruce. She moved into an austere apartment, obtained menial employment and resumed the education she had abandoned during her pregnancy in high school. She used any spare time and money to search for her daughter.

Carol and Bruce's couple relationship was severely contaminated by the actions which took place around their first pregnancy. For the most part Carol was the carrier of all that was wrong with their actions while Bruce held the reasonable and logical aspects of their decision. The burden of this split and Carol's emotional responses to the abandonment of the child were more than their relationship could bear. The emotions surrounding the original deed stifled every aspect of intimacy in their marriage until it completely consumed the relationship. At the same time the symptoms became glaringly visible, the damage had been done.

There were several family of origin factors that made this marriage vulnerable to the ravages of an extraordinary crisis. First Carol had been a devout Catholic well into her teen years and was committed to a rigid code of right and wrong. She had learned to expect that she deserved punishment for wrongdoing, and accepted it without comment. She often accepted blame for her harsh father even when she had not earned it. Her father, a career military officer, imposed rigid standards of conduct on all the four children; however, only Carol accepted it compliantly. Carol had been sensitive witness to her parent's marital relationship which provided her with a model of a self effacing woman passively submitting to a master's dominance while covertly extracting a price for docile submission. She had also been most available and willing to be drawn into marital skirmishes and was locked into most parental triangulations.

As an only child born late into the marriage of emotionally closed Irish Catholic parents, Bruce was raised to believe he had to be everything for his parents. They extracted a powerful sense of obligation from him which molded him into a compliant, dutiful son. He introjected most of their values and codes of behavior without exploring the emotional content of his life. His safety and security were found in reason and logic. He allowed Carol to express the emotions for both of them while he remained loyal to his family's avowed absence of affect. He also believed that giving up a child was wrong, but logic prevailed.

As individuals and as a couple Carol and Bruce had little natural immunity to an event that struck the core of their being. In addition, because of denial on Bruce's part and a self-fulfilling prophecy of reparation on Carol's part, the couple were unable to instigate any response to early warning signals that their relationship was being eroded. In their case the trigger event was the management of a too early pregnancy and left unattended, the aftermath of this eventually destroyed their marriage.

MARITAL PREGNANCY AND THE ABORTION CHOICE

Doris and Jack met in college and married shortly after their graduation. Both were devoted to career development and their marriage was a mutual support system for this goal. Early in the marriage Doris became pregnant. The couple wrestled with the question of what to do in light of their objectives and the situation. Jack was willing to accept the pregnancy and integrate it into their plans believing that the worst scenario would mean that they would meet their goals later than they planned. Doris was adamantly opposed to this. She believed that if Jack postponed going to law school, he never would return and also she had just obtained a much sought after job which put her in position for a stellar career path. She argued that this was not the time to have a baby. It would ruin their plan. They were financially destitute yet posed on the brink of potential success. She would not hear of an unplanned pregnancy interrupting their entire life. She told Jack that there was no way that she could tolerate this pregnancy and that she would end it no matter what he said. He finally realized that the continuance of their marriage rested in his capitulation but he could not and would not take part in any aspect of the abortion process. Doris made an appointment with a clinic and went ahead with the abortion while Jack went to pay a visit to his parents in a neighboring state.

Within the next six years, while the couple steadily marched toward financial and career success, this scene was repeated twice with no variations. Each incident became a closed, locked chapter in their lives to be noted in passing but never experienced with emotion. Then a difference occurred. Once again Doris found herself pregnant but since she was secure in her job, Jack had become a partner in a prestigious law firm, they had bought their almost dream home, and life seemed to be perfect, she decided that having a baby was appropriate. Jack, however, disagreed. His mother was terminally ill with cancer and his older sister had just discovered she had MS. Jack was overwhelmed with grief and worry and insisted that he had nothing left with which to approach impending parenthood. He argued that he wanted to be fully present for the process of pregnancy, childbirth, and parenting, and that this was not the time when he could split his feelings between grief and joy. He begged Doris to abort this pregnancy as she had so easily done before. She refused. She made it clear that if she did not complete this pregnancy, she would never have a child. She adamantly vowed to need to have a first child before she turned thirty and this was her last chance to meet her need. Jack was clear that he resented her imposing a pregnancy on him when his needs as a son and brother were so great and that should she go through with this, she could expect nothing from him as emotional support or involvement. The birth of their son and the death of Jack's mother occurred close enough to each other so that not only was he unavailable to share in the process, he had no emotional support for his loss from anyone emotionally close to him. As Doris became wrapped up in the joys of motherhood, he sequestered his grief and his resentment.

Another untimely pregnancy occurred that resulted in another abortion. This one Doris "took care of" first and informed Jack afterwards. He symbolically shrugged and went on. His experience was that anything he had to say in the realm of reproduction was futile, so why bother. Their finances were stable, they had upgraded their living situation, their careers were secure. There was nothing to prevent them from becoming parents again. Jack didn't want another child now. He wasn't sure if he ever wanted another child. However, conception was not a problem, but Doris didn't let Jack know about the pregnancy until well after a safe abortion could be performed. She wanted to spare him from having to decide or argue with her.

During this pregnancy Jack began an ill concealed affair with a co-worker. He vehemently denied Doris' suspicions and used her accusations as an excuse to be totally uninvolved with the pregnancy. There were minor complications during this pregnancy which at times led to a series of tests which could have compromised the pregnancy and precipitated much anguish on Doris' part which was heightened by Jack's cold demeanor. His position was that she wanted the pregnancy, he didn't. She kept him out of the decision process. He wanted no part of the pregnancy process.

Despite the conditions under which gestation proceeded, a healthy daughter was born. Concomitantly, Jack confessed his infidelities and the couple began couples therapy. This began a series of aborted treatment forays. Either one or the other Jack or Doris, couldn't connect with the therapist; staunchly disagreed with the process; had no respect for the techniques used. However, whenever they began with a new therapist, they rigorously supported the previous therapists and both used what a prior therapist had said or done to negate the present treatment.

Contrary to all expectations, the couple managed to garner enough from the various change agents and their processes to work toward a more mutually rewarding relationship. Jack was remorseful about the affair and Doris vowed to attempt to regain trust. In the process they were able to modify some of the more glaring interactional patterns that contributed to aspects of their marital dissatisfaction. They finally took the recommendations of their current therapist to explore some family of origin issues and other individual concerns in individual therapy while their marriage was stable enough to support this work and as there was no question about their commitment to stay married.

The fact of the abortions was denied as having any impact on their marriage by both partners. They were fervent in conveying to any therapist that these were decisions that had been made and were in the past and had no impact on the present and any persistence in pursuing the matter would only be an indication of the therapist's judgmental anti-abortion stance. The therapist, recognizing impenetrable resistance, left the matter alone believing that individual therapist with releases of information would have a more viable opportunity to touch this issues.

The couple reengaged with the marital therapist who had sent them off to individual therapy two years later. The presenting issue at this time was ironic and a parody of their past. Somehow, as a consequence of their individual therapy, they had come to a mutual decision to have a third child. Both agreed that they wanted and were ready to be co-parents. They saw the quick conception and non-threatened pregnancy as a sign that their marriage was now on firm footing. Two weeks before term, Doris delivered a still born daughter. Six months later they were both talking about ending their seventeen year marriage and a legal separation was in effect while they attempted to begin couples therapy once more.

On the surface it is inconceivable that two bright, and psychologically aware individuals could be in such complete denial about the presence of a factor with such relationship toxicity. It is not the fact of the abortion alone which infects the marriage with emotional blight, it is also in part the manner in which a deed of this magnitude is allowed to invade every aspect of relationship functioning.

The disposition for a marriage where the management of an undesirable pregnancy becomes a weapon to reenact unresolved issues grew out of family of origin factors which are beyond the scope of this article. The couple's attitude that their relationship was immune to the aftermath of a choice of the magnitude of abortion was perhaps the most unrealistic and tragic factor of all. Since their relationship remains in the realm of a "work-in-progress," there is no tidy conclusion to this case example. The prognosis is not favorable although the couple may remain technically married. They have learned to exist with the dissatisfactions of a stable and dysfunctional system. Sadly, their children may be the carriers of the aftermath of the adults' unacknowledged and therefore unresolved trauma.

Not every case that chooses abortion as a means of managing an unwelcome pregnancy is as dramatic as the one previously cited. Holly and David's circumstances are more ordinary and perhaps more typical. Their marriage was David's second, Holly's first. He had three children, 17, 19, and 23. The oldest was married with two children. Holly was a kindergarten teacher much beloved by all the children in her classes. She had ended a long-term relationship prior to meeting David and in her mid-thirties, had almost given up on getting married at all. During their dating and courtship, Holly developed a good relationship with David's children and grandchildren. Her natural connection with children was one of the traits that David found endearing. As they became more serious and intentional in their relationship, and as marriage became an option, the couple discussed the possibility of children in their joint lives. David at 48 was adamantly opposed to beginning the process of raising infants. He was content to be a grandfather. He knew that having children might be important to Holly and wanted to be clear that he would not tolerate any dissension or duplicitous breach of trust. He knew he might lose her to these conditions, yet he felt strongly enough about it to take the risk. Holly considered his words thoughtfully and with deep introspection. She looked at her life full of children in various forms, as a teacher, an aunt, a stepmother, and as a step grandmother; and she decided that she could forego the pain and pleasures of having her own biological children especially since she discovered that being a wife seemed to be more important than anything else in her life. If she had to choose between David and perhaps someday becoming a mother, she would opt for a sure thing, becoming David's wife.

The marriage progressed uneventfully for several years. They constructed a rich and meaningful relationship enhanced by their deepening interactions with David's children and their families. Shortly before Holly's fortieth birthday, she discovered that she was pregnant. At first they thought she was in early menopause, but tests confirmed that she was indeed pregnant. Without a second thought, she requested an abortion and with much emotional and physical support from David, it was carried out well before the sixth week of gestation. All went well. Holly seemed to have no regrets and David was more than understanding.

Within the next ten years, Holly became increasingly depressed, a condition that her medical doctor believes was related to the onset on menopause. Being adverse to simply prescribing medication for her, he suggested that she seek out psychotherapy prior to beginning a regime of anti-depressant drugs.

Holly's therapist spent time with her exploring possible causes for depression and in a chance remark opened the door to a closely guarded secret. The therapist observed that Holly appeared to be in the throes of grieving despite the fact that there was no actual death in her family to precipitate the bereavement reaction. The flood of tears that followed seemed completely out of proportion to the comment. However, when the crying slowed down, Holly was able to tell the therapist that indeed there had been a death that she hadn't realized was so meaningful to her and she began the process of telling the therapist about her abortion. Holly never blamed David for the abortion. She was clear that she fully agreed to the conditions he imposed. Further, she did not hesitate when confronted with the pregnancy. She realized that she would honor the terms of their contract. However, when she discovered that she was marking times and events which belonged to the child she aborted, she couldn't understand what was happening and kept the process to herself, thinking that something was wrong with her. She related to the therapist that the year her child would have been entering kindergarten was the most difficult year of her long teaching career. She had seriously contemplated leaving teaching and was barely able to complete the school year. She confessed that she marked an imaginary birthday each year and approached the anniversary of the abortion with dread in intense migraine headaches.

After the therapist had heard the extent of the "story" over several sessions, she suggested that Holly bring David into sessions to help his wife bring about a resolution. When he attended, the therapist assisted Holly in telling David her story in a non-judgmental way. David was deeply moved and disturbed that his wife had kept this to herself and had been unable to turn to him with her concerns. He was genuinely remorseful that he had unintentionally been the instrument of his wife's pain. He didn't know if he would or could have made a different decision, but he wondered what the outcome might have been if they had discussed her reluctance at the time of the abortion.

The couple realized that what might have been was no longer a viable option for them and yet at the same time they needed to find a means to somehow put the past to rest for themselves so that they could continue the remainder of their lives without such an extreme burden. They also realized that somehow the process needed to include recognition of the correctness and the wrongness of their decision about the abortion. They devised a ritual, nine months in duration, which they believed would be an act of atonement and completion. The first part of their ritual involved shopping together for a layette for a baby girl. Holly had learned, immediately following the abortion, that the child she carried was a daughter. This layette they donated to a shelter for abused women with children with the assurance that it would be used for a needy mother with a new-born daughter. The second of their ritual took them to an inner city hospital where they volunteered their time in the new-born nursery, holding and attempting to soothe infants who were born drug addicted or HIV infected. They spend three evenings a week in this capacity for almost nine months. They performed their duties together, often in tears, occasionally being able to find satisfaction in being able to comfort a very disturbed infant.

At the end of the year, on the anniversary of the abortion, they consulted a clerical person to arrange for a memorial service for their never born infant. Following that, they paid a final visit to their therapist, to let her know that they were fully finished with the secrecy of the event and with the aftermath of the event itself. They agreed that it was an accepted topic of discussion without apologies for any part of it and they related that in the process of putting it to rest, their relationship had been strengthened and the love had deepened. Holly also noted that she was able to enter into her grandmother role with David's children with greater enthusiasm and found it a rewarding interaction.

CONCLUSION

In general the therapist's awareness of the potential significance of the management of an undesired pregnancy can assist treatment in various different ways. It can keep the therapist grounded in realistic expectations. As exemplified with Doris and Jack, with their degree of denial about other factors as well as abortion, the therapist worked with what was possible without getting mired in what could not be changed. This allowed the couple to have an experience where they were neither judged nor dismissed, or chastised for being resistant. The time for meaningful change for them may still be in the future and allowing the window for treatment to remain open and available assures a genuinely positive experience in the present, which could be a prelude to greater change at another time.

These three case studies exemplify the magnitude of significance and ramification that the management of an unwelcome pregnancy presents to a couple system. However, it is not only the couple who must be prepared to confront those extraordinary conditions that are life and death issues and from which there is no turning back. The therapist must also be equipped to provide the means by which the couple may recover from the catastrophe personally and systemically intact. The first requirement to achieving this goal is an awareness of what constitutes the potential for a catastrophic event in the life of a couple. The confrontation and management of an unwelcome pregnancy with abortion or adoption constructs conditions from which a couple cannot emerge without pernicious effects. In an exploration and re-mediation of these effects, the therapist can become the instrument of repair and restoration for the partners and their relationship. It only begins, however, with the therapist's commitment to asking about abortion or adoption in a manner that encourages and supports revelation.

While both these couples confronted the circumstances of an unwelcome pregnancy with the same solution, abortion, their cases are very different. The first is dominated by covert issues and unresolved family of origin factors while the second is mostly grounded in a realistic context. In addition, therapy appeared to be unable to break through the wall of denial that shrouds of Jack and Doris, while Holly and David were open to the avenues for change. However, in both cases a knowledge of the abortion and an appreciation of the magnitude of impact of the abortion decision was helpful to the therapist. In the first case, this awareness allowed the therapist to remain consistently in the role of a conjoint expert not taking more or less responsibility for the outcome of therapy than was due. In the second case, the knowledge provided the therapist with a frame from which to work toward resolution and integration of a client's pain-filled reality.

When Your Client's Baby Dies

Deborah E. Rich

SUMMARY. Although pregnancy loss is not an uncommon occurrence, most therapists are unprepared to help clients who experience this loss. This article provides a therapist starter kit including: (1) current hospital standards of practice and services, (2) time lines for common grief reactions, (3) considering a subsequent pregnancy, (4) predictors for grief outcomes, (5) theories about the damage and recovery from perinatal loss, (6) effective therapeutic interventions and (7) issues of therapist countertransference. The entire discussion is set in a context of gender differences, i.e., how making and losing a baby is a very particular experience for each member of the couple. *[Article copies available for a fee from The Haworth Document Delivery Service: 1-800-342-9678. E-mail address: getinfo@haworthpressinc.com <Website: http://www.haworthpressinc. com>]*

KEYWORDS. Pregnancy, miscarriage, stillbirth, couple therapy, grief

When therapists think about working with pregnant clients, we ordinarily anticipate the happy outcome of the parents bringing home a healthy baby. We are honored, touched, curious, and may have a myriad of feelings activated as the pregnancy progresses. Yet, pregnancy loss, for which most therapists are unprepared, is not an uncommon occurrence. In one year in

Deborah E. Rich, MA, is a Licensed Psychologist in private practice in St. Paul, MN. She is currently completing her doctorate in counseling psychology at the University of Minnesota. Her dissertation research is on post-pregnancy loss services and grief outcome.

Address correspondence to: Deborah E. Rich, 1836 Iglehart Ave., St. Paul, MN 55104.

[Haworth co-indexing entry note]: "When Your Client's Baby Dies." Rich, Deborah E. Co-published simultaneously in *Journal of Couples Therapy* (The Haworth Press, Inc.) Vol. 8, No. 2, 1999, pp. 49-60; and: *Couples and Pregnancy: Welcome, Unwelcome, and In-Between* (ed: Barbara Jo Brothers) The Haworth Press, Inc., 1999, pp. 49-60. Single or multiple copies of this article are available for a fee from The Haworth Document Delivery Service [1-800-342-9678, 9:00 a.m. - 5:00 p.m. (EST). E-mail address: getinfo@ haworthpressinc.com].

the United States alone, according to the National Center for Health Statistics (Borg and Lasker, 1988), close to one million families experience a pregnancy loss. Out of the 3.67 million infants born alive, over 25,000 (one in 144) die during the first twenty-eight days of life and are counted as neonatal deaths. An additional 30,000 babies (about one in every 123 deliveries) are stillborn, having died between the twentieth week of pregnancy and the time of birth. The most common pregnancy failure of all is miscarriage, which is estimated to occur in fifteen to twenty percent of all recognized pregnancies, and may affect up to 900,000 families each year. In all probability, a therapist working with clients of "childbearing years," will inevitably encounter that dramatic moment of being informed that your client's baby has died.

Until the mid-1980s, there was very little professional literature about the emotional repercussions of perinatal loss. In the past ten years, two primary categories of perinatal loss literature have evolved: care providers have written anecdotally about patient experiences and clinical needs, and parents have written personal accounts of their loss and grief. While empirical literature about the short term and long term mental health repercussions of perinatal loss has increasingly appeared in the last five years, conclusions are inconsistent. Further, there is a dearth of empirical literature on effective interventions and the impact on grief outcome.

Even more striking is that the literature and service delivery remain heavily biased toward maternal attachment and maternal mourning. The inattention to the impact of perinatal loss on the father contributes to his feeling as though he is either invisible, or in contrast, solely responsible for his partner's well-being. Over time, this creates distance and strain on the couple relationship, and can lead to a relationship crisis.

The most likely circumstances in which the couple therapist will confront these issues are with ongoing clients. It is crucial that the therapist continue working with the couple rather than referring them to a specialist. This article will provide the necessary tools and information to effectively meet this challenge.

First, I will provide the basic starter kit for work with perinatal loss issues; an amalgam of my ten years of specialization in this field interwoven with the ideas of other clinicians and researchers. I will discuss the current practices and services offered to couples after pregnancy loss, time lines for common grief reactions, considerations related to subsequent pregnancies, and predictors for grief outcomes. Second, I will describe relevant theories about the nature of the damage and recovery from perinatal loss. Third, I will discuss effective therapeutic interventions and issues of therapist countertransference. The entire discussion will be set in a context of gender differences, i.e., how making and losing a baby is a very different experience for each member of the couple.

RECOMMENDED PROTOCOLS

Since the early 1980s, perinatal bereavement organizations have developed locally and nationally in an effort to meet the support needs of bereaved parents, but also to build a bridge with and educate professional caregivers. Bereavement Services/RTS (formerly known as Resolve Through Sharing) is perhaps the most prominent national organization, devoted to establishing standard protocols in hospital settings, funeral homes and for clergy of all denominations to respond to perinatal death. While there are no large scale quantitative outcome evaluations of these recommendations, they have become standard practice nationally.

In most circumstances, parents are offered the choice to see and hold their baby, even when there is an early miscarriage and tissue is not yet recognizable as human. When there is a recognizable baby, parents are encouraged to take photos and gather mementos such as a lock of hair, footprints, birth blanket and death certificate. Parents are also asked to make decisions quite quickly about baptism, naming, and burial arrangements.

Hospital protocol requires parental consent for these procedures, which can create the situation of a seemingly endless parade of people and paperwork at a time when the parents are overwhelmed. Those parents who encounter trained staff who provide written information and allow them time to think and talk privately or with chosen support people seem to fare better in the long run of the recovery process.

NORMAL TIMELINES AND REACTIONS

Swanson-Kaufmann (1986) interviewed parents who had experienced a miscarriage and found that 75% of them perceived the loss as the death of their baby. The other 25% expressed sadness about the termination of a wanted pregnancy, but did not feel attached to a baby. This paper focuses on those parents for whom the loss is experienced as the death of their baby.

While every individual and couple have a range of reactions to perinatal loss, there are common themes. Davidson (1979, 1984) proposes a four-stage model of perinatal bereavement. As with any linear model, it is important to keep in mind that stages are continuous, and that elements within a stage may be repeated in subsequent stages. This model is problematic in that it skips what is potentially a critical period of time from 9-18 months post loss, which I will discuss later. However, it serves as a useful guide for the starter kit.

Stage (1): Shock and Numbness

Shock and numbness is most intense in the first two weeks, but has recurring elements which are prominent at the anniversary date of the loss. During this stage, parents have significant difficulty concentrating and making decisions. They generally feel stunned and alternate between disbelief and feeling overwhelmed about accepting the reality of what has happened. They are being asked to make difficult and often irreversible decisions at a time when they are least capable of doing so.

Time confusion is also a common experience at this stage. Trained hospital staff are encouraged to intervene by slowing down hospital protocol as much as possible. The bereaved couple must be given information repeatedly, and important decisions should not be rushed whenever possible. In particular, the options to see and hold the baby and taking photographs should be offered many times. Staff often look to the husband to make these decisions, assuming the wife is too distraught. A husband that accepts this responsibility is caught in a dilemma of wanting to avoid burdening his wife. Yet, having made irreversible decisions which she later regrets sets the stage for future resentments which may feel insurmountable. It is very difficult for parents to resolve regrets about decisions they made at this time. Such decisions are usually the result of uncomfortable hospital staff rushing through a checklist of tasks without regard for the parents' ability to function so rapidly.

In the first few days or week, the parents are occupied with the events of medical care and funeral or disposition of the baby. Their contact with the world is quite distorted, and they are commonly isolated from their usual activities. When the initial mourning rituals are concluded, friends and family disappear, leaving the couple to fend for themselves. At this time, couples may feel utter despair over their loss and their inability to comfort themselves. The therapist meeting with a couple at this time may experience the intensity of their emotion, or may experience the couple as blunted. It is important to make explicit the normalcy of their difficulty coping.

Stage (2): Searching and Yearning

Searching and yearning is prominent from the second week through the fourth month. Themes of this stage also recur at the anniversary date of the loss. Somatic symptoms of depression and anxiety are common during this time, and must be placed in the context of normal grieving. It is at this point that gender differences in symptoms begin to emerge. Mothers commonly complain of a feeling of aching or empty arms. It is as though her body has been genetically programmed to hold the anticipated child and aches physically and emotionally due to its absence. Even though in many instances there is no known cause for the baby's death, or nothing the parents could have done to change the outcome, mothers often express feelings of guilt and self-blame. A common and effective coping mechanism is that she may need to retell the story of the pregnancy and loss repeatedly in an effort to gain mastery of the reality of the event and of her helplessness. This may appear to be a preoccupation with the deceased baby, but generally diminishes in intensity and frequency over time.

Both mothers and fathers report dreams about searching for a lost baby, and wake with a feeling of needing to find something. Whereas fathers have generally returned to work and have their daily routine to both ground and distract them, mothers are often still at home recuperating. Their isolation from familiar routine now extends to being isolated from their partner as well. The partners each develop separate coping mechanisms to handle their time apart. When the father returns home, the mother may yearn to share her intense feelings. He is generally expected to care for his partner both physically and emotionally, yet doing so places him uncomfortably close to unmanageably intense feelings. The couple begin to direct their anger about the tragic loss toward each other. A complicated dynamic ensues in which they resent the way their loss of closeness and comfort reminds them of the loss of the baby. They feel angry and helpless, and as though the only person in the world who could understand them doesn't.

Couples at this stage often have difficulty resuming physical and sexual intimacy, yet are too ashamed to bring up the subject in therapy. Engaging in sex is both a painful reminder of the tragic outcome of the pregnancy, and may feel like a betrayal of what they impose as appropriate mourning behavior. The therapist must ask them about this aspect of their relationship. This is especially critical as couples begin considering the possibility of attempting a subsequent pregnancy.

Couples will often ask for advice about the right timing to try to get pregnant again. A good landmark is the resumption of physical intimacy for the sake of closeness, comfort and pleasure. The couple who skips this step, and resumes sex only for the purpose of another pregnancy, merely complicates what is already a serious rift in the couple as an adequate family unit. Therapeutic interventions may require helping the couple relearn a repertoire of intimate verbal and physical communication.

Stage (3): Disorientation

Disorientation is prominent during the fifth to ninth month. It is during this time that the initial shock wears off. The tasks related to memorializing the baby have been completed. The nursery is disassembled. The reality of the irreversible nature of the loss emerges as an ongoing awareness. The couple feels emotionally and physically exhausted from the experience, wonders if the intensity will ever end, and has run out of things to do.

At this time, couples fear that they are deteriorating in functioning. It is important to reassure them that the intensity will subside with time. What they are experiencing is the falling away of the protective shield of shock and numbness. In addition, there is nothing more to do or say about the baby, and life must go on. This struggle of needing to let go of the intensity can be very painful. All the couple has of the relationship with the baby is the intense feelings of loss. To let go of these may feel like a betrayal, and other life events and responsibilities may pale in relative importance. As the vivid sensory memories of the events surrounding the death diminish, the couple experiences another layer of loss.

It is at this time that mementos are crucial. Parents can be encouraged to view photographs and mementos with some regularity. This activity is an opportunity for them to "be with their baby," and also gives them practice at purposefully and symbolically taking out and putting away their intense feelings and memories. Generally, parents develop a routine of visiting a grave site if there is one. An alternative is for parents to make or purchase an object that serves the purpose of the gravestone. Again, this is not a morbid activity, but an essential tool for them to master control over their feelings of loss.

At six months post loss, a critical shift in functioning generally occurs. Mothers who have received supportive care from their husbands, family and friends appear ready to adapt to life without the baby. They often become involved in activities that demonstrate their will to honor the baby by making something of their lives. Husbands, in contrast, have held their feelings at bay in order to care for their wives. Often, they mistakenly believe that they are "over" the loss. When their wives no longer need them "to be strong," they are frightened to find themselves emotionally crashing (Thomas and Striegel, 1995).

This crossover in functioning usually coincides with an intensification of the wife's desire to decide about a subsequent pregnancy. The husband may be so overwhelmed by his unexpected flood of emotions as to be unable to consider this decision. The couple therapist must help the couple pace their emotional dependence on each other. In addition, a thoughtful discussion about the meaning of a subsequent pregnancy illuminates each of their true motives, desires and fears. The couple may not have previously examined the pregnancy decision, and will need help negotiating new territory.

It is at this point that Davidson's model is inadequate. He skips over the crucial period of 9-18 months post loss when the couple face many anniversary dates: the due date, the date of conception, the date of the loss, and all the anticipated first holidays and events. Complicating matters is that issues surrounding a subsequent pregnancy are prominent at this time, and strain the couples ability to both memorialize the baby who died and prepare for a new child. The couple may be experiencing difficulty getting pregnant or may already be pregnant. It is helpful to normalize the couple's fears about experiencing another loss in the form of infertility, or another death.

The therapist must also be mindful of helping the couple begin to attach to the new baby, preventing the dynamic of a replacement child. Specifically, it is advisable for them to select new names for the next child. While they may choose to keep some special gifts that were intended for the baby who died, it is also advisable for them to provide tangible cues that this is a different child, for example, new clothes, bedding and toys.

Stage (4): Reorganization/Resolution

Reorganization/resolution emerges between 18-24 months post loss. During this stage, the couple generally experiences a sense of release from the intensity of loss. They are able to function adequately with normal daily routines. DeFrain (1986) conducted a retrospective study of nearly 500 couples who had experienced a stillborn child. These couples reported that by two years post loss they were able to *function* as well as prior to the loss. However, a significant number of couples reported that a return to the *previous level of happiness* took 5-7 years post loss. As with any retrospective study, there are limits of generalizability, however, in another retrospective study, Lehman (1986) found similar results. There were no significant gender differences in long term functioning in either of these studies.

Lasker and Toedter (1991) conducted a five-year longitudinal study which included 138 pregnancy losses. Approximately half of the male partners also participated in the study which evaluated bereaved parents for three categories of grief outcomes: active grief, difficulty coping and despair. Parents were evaluated at three time periods post-loss: 6-8 weeks, 12 months, and 25-29 months. Lasker and Toedter (1991) found that gestational age (the longer the pregnancy, the more active grief), parent gender (women higher than men), strength of the couple relationship, and expectancy of problems (from conclusive medical evidence) were significant factors in active grief outcomes. Two smaller studies found similar results (Conway and Valentine, 1987; Theut et al., 1989). Surprisingly, previous mental health functioning alone was not a reliable predictor of active grief outcome.

In Lasker and Toedter's (1991) study, significant gender differences also included that women scored higher than men on guilt and anger, and one third of the women studied felt they were to blame for the child's death even though there was no medical evidence to indicate this. However, when looking at difficulty coping outcome, men and women were comparable. Quality of physical health, supportive friends and having living children were helpful factors in coping with grief (Lasker and Toedter, 1991; Theut et al., 1989). The experience of previous losses had inconclusive impact on grief in the first year post loss, but stood out in impact on functioning in subsequent years.

Finally, men, particularly from lower social classes, scored higher on despair than did women. In fact, there were three suicide attempts among study subjects, all men (Lasker, 1990). One could speculate that women's process of active grief was a palliative factor in grief outcome, and that therapist interventions with bereaved fathers should incorporate education and encouragement about expressing grief.

THERAPEUTIC FRAMEWORKS

Therapeutic frameworks for understanding uncomplicated perinatal be-reavement are significantly more elaborate in describing maternal than paternal mourning. From a developmental perspective, reproduction is both a biological capacity and a developmental task (Brice, 1982; Davidson, 1990; Leon, 1990). Culturally determined childbearing years are essentially the critical period during which individuals and couples grapple with the personal meaning of having children. Generally, women derive a measure of self-esteem from the successful accomplishment of this developmental task. The experience of in-fertility or perinatal loss presents developmental interference resulting in nar-cissistic injury (Leon, 1990). A more complicated developmental perspective suggests that early developmental themes of separation and individuation play a role in the development of feelings of shame and guilt (Davidson, 1990). The failure to reproduce essentially activates themes of separation and individua-tion, i.e., successful achievement of adulthood, and initiates a domino effect whereby the pregnancy loss activates previous unresolved losses each with their attendant feelings of shame and guilt. While this is helpful in understand-ing the apparent irrational experience of maternal self-blame, it offers no clues about the father's developmental crisis. One can only speculate about the roles of virility and fertility in male self-esteem. Clearly since men are not capable of carrying a pregnancy, their experience of personal responsibility for a success-ful pregnancy is quite different from the woman.

Many couples struggle with the inequities in responsibility for and the accompanying trade-offs in bonding with the unborn child. The husband may feel cheated that he was unable to have any physical closeness with the unborn child. Yet, that same husband may also feel guilty that his wife has to suffer what feels to him to be a greater loss. The therapist must balance the unique and different experiences for the husband and wife, while helping them to avoid quantifying and comparing their relative experience of the loss. Our society is so focused on maternal-infant bonding, that fathers generally lack a vocabulary to describe the meaning to them of producing and of losing a child.

Brice (1991) took a fascinating approach to perinatal bereavement. He strongly disagreed with the usefulness of a stage model, and instead con-ceptualized five paradoxes of maternal mourning which present an ongoing

existential-phenomenological struggle for the bereaved mother. For the couple therapist, being familiar with the content of these paradoxes and the
unresolvable nature of the dilemmas provides a useful framework for the
therapeutic work.

Paradoxes of World Transformation

For the newly bereaved parent, the child's death essentially feels like the
death of the world as they know it. The parents develop a vigilant awareness
of other deaths and births, and are faced with the divergence of their life
experience from the normal order of things. The dilemma for parents is to
choose to go on living when perhaps the only way to join the child would be
through death. Symbolically, parents represent a choice to go on living when
they renew old interests, or are compelled into new ones. It is as if they
commit to live life to the fullest in order to honor the memory of the baby.

Paradoxes of Relating to the Child

The parents' mental images of the child or dreamed for child are in sharp
contrast to the absence of that child. While they have empty arms, so to
speak, they are full of grief. For a period of time, the only way they have of
relating to the child is to immerse themselves in the grief feelings. The
dilemma for parents is to resolve the paradox of maintaining a relationship
with the dead child by creating an unreal live child who is the recipient of
their intense longing.

Paradoxes of Self-Deception

The newly bereaved parent experiences a continuous existence between
disbelief and acceptance. They may continue searching for an explanation
when all avenues are exhausted, and no information is adequate. They perpetu-
ate the child's existence through child-related projects. While this is an effective coping mechanism, as mentioned earlier, it becomes a dilemma when the
parent runs out of things to do. Unfortunately some bereaved parents rely on
distractions such as trips away, drugs, or impulsive behavior; but they don't
last. Finally, parents need to understand the paradox that momentarily feeling
good and being better are not equivalent. It is important not to rush bereaved
parents into reporting being better than they know they are.

Paradoxes of Responsibility and Unfairness

Mothers particularly feel inordinate responsibility for the baby's death,
and experience the paradox of guilt, caught between actual helplessness and

the myth of maternal omnipotence. In addition, bereaved parents look at the babies around them and feel envious and jealous. They find reasons why other people don't deserve live babies, "How can crack addicted moms produce healthy babies?" or, "Why should that teenager have irresponsible sex and then get a healthy baby when we have planned and have the maturity to care for a child?" While they know it is irrational and even cruel to wish others' babies dead, they struggle with the unfairness of pregnancy outcomes.

Paradoxes of Interpersonal Relations

Each member of the couple desperately needs a listening other, yet since their experiences, feelings and needs are different, they can grow to resent each other both for being needy and for being an inadequate comfort. At the same time, they are ambivalent about talking with others. In spite of this, the hellish experience often brings increased capacity for compassion and understanding of others, and hopefully eventually of each other. The prominent dilemma is that while getting over the intensity of early grief means feeling better, it also means forgetting the child. The parents are unable to avoid the conflict between resisting and surrendering to the healing process.

TREATMENT RECOMMENDATIONS

According to Leon (1987), 75% of bereaved parents want to discuss the loss. Clinically, he found a statistically significant decrease in depression and anxiety for those parents receiving supportive counseling, and believed that to be the treatment of choice. He argued that the developmental interference of failed pregnancy may be exacerbated by the regressive process of intensive therapy. Brice (1982), a psychoanalyst, suggested that it is a serious mistake for clinicians to emphasize only the here-and-now ego state of the mourner and ignore past developmental issues. For therapists of any orientation, what is most important is to place the loss in the context of the personal histories of the parents.

The treatment can be thought of as a journey. The therapist together with the clients fully explore the complexities of the mourning world, including irrational guilt and fantasies. The therapist engages the couple in active inquiry, and is emotionally responsive as they debrief. The therapist also stands on firm ground, infusing fact and reality into the therapeutic experience.

While couple therapy can be extremely helpful, and should not be disrupted by the occurrence of a pregnancy loss, perinatal bereavement support groups should also be considered. A well run couples group dealing with perinatal bereavement enables the couple to discover that they are not alone in their experience or their feelings. It also offers them a break from needing to be attentive and understanding with each other; it diffuses the intensity between them. Another grieving couple who is farther ahead in the healing process can be enormously reassuring for the newly bereaved couple wondering how they will survive this loss. In many such groups, husbands are customarily motivated to attend merely to accompany and support their wives. Once attending regularly, however, they develop a comfort and a vocabulary to express their own individual experience. It cannot be overemphasized that for men, the modeling and support of other bereaved fathers is a critical ingredient in their recovery.

THERAPIST CONSIDERATIONS

Listening to the tragic stories of bereaved parents can be difficult. It often revives old losses for the therapist, and forces them to face their own response to death. It is understandable for the therapist to wish to rescue the parents, to make things better, to offer concrete actions, or to overidentify and overdisclose. It is essential for the therapist to resist these urges, as well as the one to refer out.

Consider this an opportunity for self-reflection, perhaps incorporating this professional struggle into your own therapy work. This is only, after all, a life-cycle event; a normal developmental passage that has a tragic outcome. Certainly effective therapy involves the ability to help clients embrace such life circumstances even as we struggle to do so ourselves.

REFERENCES

Borg, S. and Lasker, J. (1988). *When pregnancy fails: Families coping with miscarriage, ectopic pregnancy, stillbirth, and infant death.* Boston: Beacon Press.

Brice, C.W. (1982). Mourning throughout the life cycle. *American Journal of Psychoanalysis*, 42(4), 315-325.

Brice, C.W. (1991). Paradoxes of maternal mourning. *Psychiatry*, 54(1), 1- 12.

Conway, P. and Valentine, D. (1987). Reproductive losses and grieving. *Journal of Social Work and Human Sexuality*, 6(1), 43-64.

Davidson, C. (1990). *Shame and guilt and the experience of bereavement.* Paper delivered to the National Perinatal Bereavement Association bi-annual meeting, Atlanta, GA, October, 1990.

Davidson, G.W. (1979). *Understanding death of the wished for child.* Springfield, IL: OGR Service Corporation.

Davidson, G.W. (1984). *Understanding mourning.* Minneapolis: Augsburg Publishing House.

DeFrain, J. (1986). *Stillborn: The invisible death.* Lexington, MA: Lexington Books.

Lasker, J.H. (1990). *Weaving grief into the fabric of life.* Paper delivered to the National Perinatal Bereavement Association bi-annual meeting, Atlanta, GA, October, 1990.

Lasker, J.H., and Toedter, L.J. (1991). Acute vs. chronic grief: The case of pregnancy loss. *American Journal of Orthopsychiatry*, 61, 510-522.

Lehman, D.R., Ellard, J.H., and Wortman, C.B. (1986). Social support for the bereaved: Recipients' and providers' perspectives on what is helpful. *Journal of Consulting and Clinical Psychology*, 54(4), 438-446.

Leon, I.G. (1987). Short term psychotherapy for perinatal loss. *Psychotherapy*, 24(2), 186-195.

Leon, I.G. (1990). *When a baby dies: Psychotherapy for pregnancy and newborn loss.* New Haven, CO: Yale University Press.

Swanson-Kauffman, K.M. (1986). Caring in the instance of unexpected early pregnancy loss. *Topics in Clinical Nursing*, 8(2), 37-46.

Theut, S.K., Pedersen, F.A., Zaslow, M.J., Cain, R.L. et al. (1989). Perinatal loss and parental bereavement. *American Journal of Psychiatry*, 146(5), 635-639.

Thomas, V. and Striegel, P. (1995). Stress and grief of a perinatal loss: Integrating qualitative and quantitative methods. *Journal of Death and Dying*, 30(4), 299-311.

Men and Post-Abortion Grief: Amendment, Resolution and Hope

E. Mark Stern

SUMMARY. This article highlights the nub of psychotherapy done with three men suffering from the emotional ravages of interrupted pregnancies. It demonstrates, through clinical descriptions, the effects of post-abortion grief with these would-have-been-fathers. The article briefly telescopes the possibilities of helping these individuals create new foundations for their own survival. *[Article copies available for a fee from The Haworth Document Delivery Service: 1-800-342-9678. E-mail address: getinfo@haworthpressinc.com <Website: http://www.haworthpressinc.com>]*

KEYWORDS. Pregnancy, abortion, men, grief, loss

Whose name is called He-is-with-us
because he did not abhor the uterus
Whereby these uteral forms
are to us most dear

–William Blake,
Jerusalem, *pl. 7. I: 65*

POST-ABORTION GRIEF

Although it has become routine to accept "life" as the continuum which follows birth, prevailing linear reasoning is hard pressed to declare the "ex-

E. Mark Stern, EdD, ABPP, is Professor Emeritus, Graduate Faculty of Arts and Sciences, Iona College.

Address correspondence to: E. Mark Stern, 215 East Eleventh Street, New York, NY 10003.

[Haworth co-indexing entry note]: "Men and Post-Abortion Grief: Amendment, Resolution and Hope." Stern, E. Mark. Co-published simultaneously in *Journal of Couples Therapy* (The Haworth Press, Inc.) Vol. 8, No. 2, 1999, pp. 61-71; and: *Couples and Pregnancy: Welcome, Unwelcome, and In-Between* (ed: Barbara Jo Brothers) The Haworth Press, Inc., 1999, pp. 61-71. Single or multiple copies of this article are available for a fee from The Haworth Document Delivery Service [1-800-342-9678, 9:00 a.m. - 5:00 p.m. (EST). E-mail address: getinfo@haworthpressinc.com].

act" moment a fetus actually "becomes" a human creature. Because of a failure to adequately determine *what* life shall be mourned, society often downplays the possibility of a man's grief following the abortion of an embryo or fetus he had fathered. Over the span of a 40 plus year practice, it has come to my attention that, following the termination of a pregnancy, a significant number of would-have-been fathers have suffered a variety of reactions, ranging from fear of failure, profound loss, moral anguish and/or a sense of personal bodily mutilation.

Post-abortion grief in men can result in a chronic depression during which sleep disturbances and nightmares are not uncommon. Complicating these reactions is the all but impossible often found incapacity to cry or otherwise vent feelings that may be gutted by hidden guilt and sorrow.

It matters little whether the would-have-been-father had consented to the abortion. Those whose religious backgrounds stress the sacredness of nascent life may be prone to view the destruction of a living fetus as a breach of a covenant with God. Men who claim to be neutral or even positive about abortion are hardly immune from unrelenting bouts of sadness and regret.

Abortion is the elective destruction of a fetus. This process can be experienced by some men as a threat to the continuity of their own lives: those who literally despair of having lost their own destinies. Here denial of personal responsibility is crucial. Incompetence and shame mesh in with feticide motifs, resulting in alienation, psychic numbing and suicidal fantasies.

JOHN

John lamented long after the abortion. His continuing bouts of middle-of-the-night anxiety awakened him from corrosive images of star-shaped and stunted fetuses. These nocturnal onslaughts haunted his days. He avoided social situations which reminded him of newborns and children.

John shamed Eliza for having had the abortion. Although their relationship would ultimately improve, there was little to hide the fact that an impenetrable wall existed between them. John felt alone. He referred to himself as "the other victim" of the abortion. Anger, grief and morbidity overwhelmed him. Yet these emotional wounds eventually allowed him to sift through and enlarge on his own values. Above all else he loved Eliza.

Through all of John's shaming insinuations, Eliza remained steadfast in her devotion to him. John, in his way, wanted to forgive if not forget. Eliza, according to him, had been a victim of an overenthusiastic worker in a woman's health center.

Eliza did what she could to rally her support against John's morbidity. "Listen to me you damn fool," she blurted, "abortion was my only option," and: "John, speak the truth, were so ready to commit to a baby? I know that you would have hated the imposition. . . . (Pause) And now, at least, we don't have to make hasty decisions about the future."

Eliza's outspokeness was sometimes comforting, though hardly enough for John. John felt betrayed and grief ridden. The recurring nightmares impinged upon his sleep. When questioned about his moods, he spoke of being driven to a kind of death. Both realized that a special vitality been lost between them. John sought therapy for himself.

I suggested that John draw sketches of the unborn child. When I asked him to comment on them, he was quick to point to a parent and child arrangement: "Something like the dead figure on the mother's lap in Michelangelo's *Pieta*."

I asked him to try to "converse" with his sketch. "If the suffering Mary is your measure," I commented, "then a conversation could well be a devotional act." There were other drawings: "Like a father joining his child at play." A shift occurred. John's drawings turned bleak and cadaverous. He finally referred to "the stunted baby I'm now carrying in my soul."

Since the abortion John had become emotionally incapable of setting his eyes on his sister's two young sons. They were painful reminders of a "might-have-been-child." John's characteristic mode was an avoidant one. The thought of visiting his nephews had become humiliating. In his eyes, he had "failed" to be what he ought to have been. John was on continuous watch, stating that if he were to ease his guard that he would become subject to outside derision as much as to inside grief. There was no "security" in his life. No way of being "connected." He cried when he spoke of Eliza, but hadn't as yet associated his tears with the lurking anger he was yet to explore.

In a landmark dream several months into his therapy, John saw himself as a patron of a small beach concession whose proprietors were a bleak young couple. Early in the dream, John ordered a hamburger. The couple responded by scrounging around for bits of "fuzzy" meat. He was anxious that ingredients be found and put together properly.

The scene shifted. John was now what appeared several miles down the beach. He envisioned a man walking with his four year old young son. John was amazed at how well matched they were. He looked on in envy. Suddenly an old friend from high school took shape. This friend Alec, had in fact, died of cancer two years earlier. In the dream, he was John's long-lost buddy. Suddenly, John found himself baby-sitting the four year old who he "recognized" as Alec's son.

John woke up with an "aftertaste" of the dream. He was amazed at the dream's lucidity. Associations flowed: The bare larder was comparable to his situation with Eliza. "That couple could have been us struggling with our confusion." Qualms about something/someone (he later saw the "fuzzy" meat as the disassembled embryo) *missing* became the mainstay of his postdream terror. Through it all, he wondered if the couple were simply stand-ins for his "poor" relationship with Eliza. Financial insecurity, he told himself, was a strong factor in deciding on the abortion. He recalled that prior to their going to the abortion clinic, Eliza had said, "Babies need to be fed." John felt accused of not being able to scrounge up "the necessary bucks" to feed a family. Later he extended his view of poor as signifying constant uncertainty and disharmony in the marriage.

John had been a faithful friend to Alec. They had known one another since ninth grade. He regularly visited Alec in his final months. "Alec looked like a baby as he was getting close to death." The dying friend and the dead fetus became homoerotically unified in the dream. The dual loss highlighted John's sense of loneliness and abandonment.

Although rebuffed by John, Eliza did what she could to waken their present. His negative mode of coping cast her in the role of "appeaser." To some degree, John idealized his grieving, even as he longed to be released from its intensity. More important was his need to appreciate the fullness of his experience. Only in his reverence for *all* that he felt regarding the loss of *their* unborn child could John's mourning represent his effort at resurrecting his relationship with Eliza. This was his paradox. His dedication to the memory of an unborn son could never be realized by aborting his responsibility to his wife.

John's therapy became a place for him to reckon with his confusion and with his enmeshment in non-being and loss. Early in our sessions I informed John that I was not there to prioritize his goals. But in the course of his therapy John did *decide* to re-establish his relationship with his nephews. The ensuing reconciliation was John's prelude to reaffirming his future with Eliza.

Therapy allowed John to face his fears of abandonment. Unearthing the deeper dynamics of such terror required steadfast dedication to the therapy. In time his productive capacities were set into motion and John began to shift his attention from extinction to making new life possible. My function, as his therapist, was to reverence his experiences: the lures of death and non-being and his growing sense of connectedness. In this way, John allowed himself to give birth to new living options.

MARTIN

Martin "ached" for the return of the aborted child he admitted to never having actually wanted. He grew increasingly furious with Gilda for having terminated her pregnancy. But he was no less enraged at himself for his failure to not "insist" that Gilda carry the baby to term. His acknowledged his confusion as the reason for his "lack of force" with Gilda. His "weakness" resulted in overwhelming self-blame. But to blame himself was to criticize Gilda even more. She found herself in a "no-win" trap.

Gilda remained confounded by Martin's "true" motives. She claimed that her decision to abort grew out of the fear that doing otherwise would be the final straw in ending their troubled relationship. Martin was indeed unclear about the value of continuing the marriage. "Some days," he said, "it feels like I'm playing the role of the woman and she the man. It's those times that I feel most abandoned by her. It's then that I drown in my confusion."

Gilda concluded that it was pointless to not "start over again." She wondered about her responsibility in helping to rehabilitate Martin's lonely past. Yet in the face of Martin's continuing accusations aimed at her, their situation seemed all the more precarious. "No," she admitted, she probably would not have done it all that differently. Yes, she would have had the abortion.

As her own therapy continued, Gilda began to learn that "simply pleasing Martin" could ultimately become self-abnegating. Years of comprising her spontaneity had taken its toll. It was true that "the reason" she had the abortion was her fear that, despite his vigorous protestations to the contrary, Martin would "leave (her) flat." She alone regretted that she might not being able to conceive a second time.

Martin was angered by Gilda's "claim to never-ending entitlements" and to her "complete ignorance of any consequences the abortion might have had on (him)." But Martin appeared to be unaware of how rampantly his narcissism projected itself onto Gilda. Gilda, according to Martin, was too much like his mother. Martin both feared and was attracted to "demanding" women of his mother's ilk. Gilda attributed her aggressivity to having survived the ravages of an alcoholic father. Her mother hardly survived. Gilda needed to know she counted, but she had little to go on. She did want a baby at that point, but "Yes, but even more than the baby," she indicated that she was not prepared "to collapse as her mother had" before her.

Despite their current conflicts, Gilda was fiercely protective of Martin. It was of significance to both she and Martin that she had been her father's "guardian till the day (he) died." Many of the dynamics in the earlier father-daughter relationship seemed to be replaying. And once again, she feared for her own life.

Martin's rages were galloping and loud. He continued to make mean-spirited accusations with little thought for their consequences. He felt much "like a ruined woman." Even his "flabby flesh" reminded him of his indeterminate body. Gilda's "flat chestedness" contributed to his restlessness and uncertainty. "She's a tough cookie, that one, and in a woman's body."

For all his noise and recriminations, Martin was himself bound up in confusing personal issues of sexual identity. He struggled with crippling memories of his mother's grandiosity and "vindictive" independence. Time and again, she had left him alone and isolated. She raged out her endless monologues, embarrassing him in front of others. He felt shamed before his contemporaries, yet felt compelled to apologize to his mother for having caused her so many problems.

Therapy took several turns before Martin was to understand that he had much to deal before he could ever come to terms with Gilda. His moods veered. One hour could be filled with severity, while the next with tenderness. Each mood served to mask the other. Yet each, in its unique way, represented veiled cries of anguish. Clearly, Martin felt unheard by his mother, and now by his wife.

Martin's mother and wife, each in their turn, would not understand why Martin was "such a sensitive person." He, in turn, experienced their aggressivity as withdrawals of support when he needed them most. Martin, even as he rejected the prospect of a baby, regarded the abortion as a way of being denied the love and support he felt he "deserved." He was dependent and vulnerable. He quaked before his fear of never becoming a father. But in the end, Martin feared most for his image and of not appearing capable and robust under all circumstances. This image, he felt, had been impeded by the abortion. Nevertheless his anger was translated into endless blame. Eventually, all of the accusations boomeranged, leaving him even more confused about his progressive disengagement from Gilda.

Martin likened his life to his brother. Steve, two years younger than Martin had twice been married and divorced. Some years before, Steve had been an exchange student in Europe. Soon after he returned to the United States, he received a letter from an ex-girlfriend. She wrote to tell him that she was pregnant with his child. Steve "agonized over the situation" for several days before advising her that it would be best for both of them if she had an abortion, Later she confessed that she had lied about being pregnant in hopes that Steve would offer to marry her.

Martin remembered the day the "all clear" arrived from Europe. But unlike Steve's recollection of being relieved, Martin vividly remembered Steve admitting to some sadness when he realized that he had not "succeeded" in impregnating the young woman. Martin related this to his own post-abortion "failure." A foiled pregnancy made' him a "failed" man.

The brothers were close. Steve advised Martin to get a divorce. Martin knew that Steve was overreacting to memories of their mother's "bitchy" controls. In the light of that control, their father never seemed to have had "much of a chance." Martin regarded his father as "an unknown all of his life." He was amiable enough; served as a Little League coach; was a moderately successful rare coin dealer and appeared to be liked by the neighbors. Yet at home he was seen as "howling in defeat" after many hours of criticisms from his wife. He was a "haunted man." In his late teens he had been a member of motorcycle cult. There were whispers of his participation in a racially motivated riot during which a black man had been stabbed to death.

Martin suspected that his father "had served (prison) time" before marriage. Silence and fading tattoos were the only surreal cues to his father's "failure." His mother would say nothing about the incident after his father's death.

Nothing seemed enough to counter Martin's distrust. Despite Gilda's reassurances, Martin's frustrated confusion had effectively frozen her out of their relationship. Lovemaking had become awkward since the abortion. Martin appeared to be inscribing his father's biography in his own life. As he became more self-justifying, Gilda found herself wanting to protect what little personal regard she had. This was not easy. Repetitions of parental rages flooded her consciousness. Life with Martin had become part of these unbearable horror stories. Although not consciously premeditated, the formula of "no sex, no children" became their articulation of a failed marriage.

Martin mourned his lost fatherhood along with the rage at the loss of his own little known father. Anguish collided with hope and possibility. Happily, in his therapy, Martin had come to regard that there was something to be learned from the worst of his experiences. Gilda was finally gone. He mourned her loss as he did the aborted baby. But even more importantly, he began to accept that her actions, included the abortion, were intrinsic by-products of her overwhelming pain. He recognized that he was far from a passing figure in Gilda's decision to abort. In part, he recognized himself as one of its active initiators. His slow recovery related well to a growing forgiveness for the wrongs done to them and by them.

PHILIP

Philip stated that he would have given his life for the survival of the aborted fetus. Death-imagery was a constant companion. His own early survival had been nip-and-tuck. He was the archetypal delicate asthmatic child. Philip referred to his existence as a combination of deadly memories. He vividly recalled the difficult battles of "reaching for breath" in the middle of the night. In his early teens, an aunt casually mentioned how his mother's plans to have had him aborted had been thwarted. "I've never felt quite real," he declared.

Philip distrusted his ability to finish projects or to appear credible in conversations. Overwhelming distractedness reinforced repeated stalemates in social relationships and working situations. He looked younger than his years and learned to affect a "innocent" boyishness. Because of his awkwardness, he'd all but given up on the hope of meeting a woman. But as the fates would have it, he did meet Kimberly in a charismatic prayer group he had recently started to attend. The group attracted a large number of singles from a wide range of educational and social backgrounds.

As Philip recalled their initial encounter, Kimberly looked vaguely uncomfortable in her ill matching outfit. Her hair was tousled from the March winds. Philip was quick to notice an ageless weathered quality about her. He thought to himself that this was the sort of woman with whom he could feel vaguely comfortable.

It turned out that Kimberly was hardly older than Philip's 24 years. Her own childhood had been largely affectionless. Her parents, who lived in a distant city, remained inflexible and censorious. They had no sympathy for Kimberly's growing religiosity nor did they show any interest in her upcoming marriage to Philip. They appeared to be betrayed and embarrassed by her marginality. And aside from the one visit they made prior to her marriage, they never again appeared while the couple remained together.

Philip described his mother as a drab little figure who built a life out of hundreds of small details. Her self-sacrificing demeanor was the only support Philip had ever known. She died while he was on the borders of failing out of college. His father had been no help at all. He had been little than a distant presence who continued to share the family house with his wife's older sister. This was the aunt who told Philip about his mother's plan to have him aborted. Father and aunt maintained a shallow relationship with Philip. Philip was convinced that his aunt had always been jealous of his mother.

Prior to and into the marriage itself, the charismatic prayer group had become the couple's surrogate family. But what meaningful contact there might have briefly been between Philip and Kimberly had since deteriorated. He had ceased attending the meetings while Kimberly relied heavily on the group's support.

Philip could not sort out why he had ever been attracted to her. Then again he was concerned that she was the only "sort of woman" that would ever be attracted to him. Philip spoke angrily about Kimberly's always being out of kilter. Nevertheless, Kimberly became pregnant less than a year into the marriage. She knew that the pregnancy was unsafe for her. She was convinced that she had made a big mistake and that Philip was an unlikely father. A weak Philip who barely spoke to her in a civil tone produced difficulties beyond repair.

Small tasks continued to be major undertakings for Philip. And the more Kimberly showed anger and disappointment, the greater did his otherwise inner-directed rage turn outward. He had lied to her about having finished college, when in truth incompletes and failing grades riddled his transcript. He attempted to get work in an office job, but routinely undermined his interviews. In a gesture typical of him, Philip would smile as he threw up his arms and spoke about the ways in which he always found himself sidelined. His "boyishness" appealed to one or another boss who tended to lighten his responsibilities. He worked in ground maintainance in a local school. The school's custodian had effectively become his custodian. But his job was by no means ever secure.

The prayer group continued its vigil on the couple's behalf, even though it was only Kimberly who still attended the weekly meetings. She had become close to an older couple whose appeared to be indispensable to her. But as time went on, even they could not furnish her with any helpful advice on how to emotionally survive in the marriage. Philip became a caricature of her parents constantly blaming her. Whereas before, she had felt enlivened by his boyishness, now she had become overwhelmed with his inability to take any responsibility for anything related to their survival.

Philip had indeed taken to his shell. And almost miraculously on the day she announced that she had decided to have an abortion, his boyishness seemed to cease. Hanging midway between terror and depression, she explained that it was all too ambiguous for her to be having a child. The couple in the prayer group had been excited by the prospect of her bearing a child. But they too could hardly lend her any meaningful support. That day proved to be catastrophic for the marriage. In the weeks that followed, the prayer group too pulled back.

Kimberly moved out. Philip became inconsolable. He seemed to forget how unmanageable the marriage had been. For him, all that remained was the memory of being thwarted once again; this time by the loss of a child. His world had become a *"might-have-been."* He claimed to be very lonely even as he avoided facing his role in the abortion. Still, as time passed, the idea of new relationships remained threatening. Philip was all the more the lost frightened child. He had moved into an embarrassed agoraphobic retreat.

Therapy helped him to get in touch with some faint awareness of shared responsibility for the abortion. He dreamt of subterranean images where the aborted child continued to exist. As time went on this dream presence became an aid to his gathering together some few emotional reserves. He had always been the fetus. The aborted fetus and the asthmatic child paralleled each other. In his dreams and imagery, together they yearned for breath and breath.

Listening to Philip's sad situation brought me back to an early episode in my own life. I had just reached my seventh year when I developed an intense infection in one of my ears. Some years before the discovery of antibiotics, the doctors had given up hope for my survival. I weighed a scarce 35 pounds as I continued to run an unusually high fever. The pain had become intolerable and chances of my pulling through major surgery were discounted. My mother, fearing the worst, went into denial and eloped to a second marriage. She had temporarily lost contact with me and had not known of my survival. For a time, she failed to mention my existence to her new husband.

I have never forgotten the weariness brought on by the unflinching pain. In the worst of this discomfort, I had little desire for life. I recall how my arms and legs were strapped into place in the operating room. The nurse-anesthetist minimized the death-hurtling effect the ether had on my very being. The noxious odor and the sensation of spinning into oblivion have remained potent memories through these many years. Perhaps these sensations of my body being forced into dismantlement reflected pre-conscious impressions of an abortion my mother had originally planned but finally opted to not have?

At an opportune moment, I told my story to Philip. He allowed that he was not alone in his grief. Our work seemed to proceed well from that point on. Philip's psychotherapy became more available to him because of my sensitivity to his pain. As two wounded fellow-travellers, we were able to skillfully relate to the forebodings of his current life. This phenomenon pushed well beyond Freudian notions of transference. Who we both were in our respective pains provided him with a place to mourn the lost fetus. This new context allowed Philip to "come forth," from his stasis, and to find remorse in his soul for the egotism and cruelty which went untended in his marriage. Philip was his own helpless babe, but within his own non-life had unwittingly helped create a circumstance where a baby did not get born. It was appropriate that he mourn all his losses. His marriage was well beyond reconciliation. Still an over-concern with the destructive tempestuousness in himself would have only prejudiced him against himself. The lost child who had been spurned was ultimately no different from his own sense of feeling alienated. He might have simply accepted his failures. Instead Philip began to work on how not to be complacent. Even the dead can contribute positively to those who survive them. In the end Philip decided that he needed to become worthy of the child who might well have been.

FINAL REFLECTIONS

Therapy styled to help men who grieve the loss of aborted children provides motivation to survive. Psychotherapy, among other things, wakens lingering grief. Such grievings have qualitative value where emotions can too easily be numbed in the name of technological accommodation. "Cures" for grief have become products in today's commodity-driven "medicalized" culture. But grieving for an unborn offspring can be more valuable than not grieving.

Post-abortion grief is a viable predicament. It can exist in both genders, though it is probably never experienced in the same way by any two people. The likelihood of a quick or even sure resolution is not to be expected. Denying the roles that grief plays in anyone's life leads to never feeling appropriately responsive. Therefore it would appear that such denial prevents a might-have-been father from ever taking any real responsibility for the denial of another person's existence.

Personal histories have a tendency to converge. Thus the goal of all personal responsibility must be a sense that relationships are worth seeing through; and that everything that has been alive or has had some chance of coming alive together with everyone who ever will be alive in any one person's life determines the focus of that life. Together people adopt each other's purposes for being. The larger repetoire of being includes grieving as a positive potentiality. Lost or unborn children symbolize lost hopes in need of reemerging as new possibilities.

The experience of post-abortion loss often eludes the detection of the behavioral scientist. No two might-have-been fathers or mothers wince in the same way. Caring, though not necessarily, curing, those who mourn keeps faith with appropriating the sacredness and individuality of grief. It is most probably in the psychotherapeutic engagement that the therapist's full presence and attention serves as a life-giving link to the reality of the who that is lost to both mother and father. And it is in the careful considerations of mourning the unborn that humanity engages in reawakening itself to the dreams it has misplaced, but has never really lost.

Of Breasts and Men:
Three Generations of Vampire Coupling

Gerald Schoenewolf

SUMMARY. This study focuses on a certain mode of relating that is apparently passed on from generation to generation. This mode, which is termed "vampire coupling," is characterized by a passive-aggressive struggle in which each member of a couple frustrate each other's oral needs for nurturing. The study describes a case history which illustrates this mode, and traces it back three generations. It also looks at the vampire myth in general and links it to the fantasies of dysfunctionally passive males. *[Article copies available for a fee from The Haworth Document Delivery Service: 1-800-342-9678. E-mail address: getinfo@haworthpressinc. com <Website: http://www.haworthpressinc.com>]*

KEYWORDS. Passive-aggression, oral-sadism, nurturing, vampire-coupling

"I was in an ambulance and I was dead. Lying beside me was a black girl and she was still alive. I took a syringe and stuck it into her neck and sucked out her blood. She died and I came alive. Then I was at my mother's house. She was there with some of her women friends. I did the same thing to them, sucked out all their blood, and they died and I lived."

This is not the dream of a vampire, but of a patient whose childhood

---

Gerald Schoenewolf, PhD, is a Practicing Psychoanalyst and Director of The Living Center, a cooperative specializing in working with artists. He is also Adjunct Associate Professor at the New York Institute of Technology and the author of eleven books, most recently *The Dictionary of Dream Interpretation*.

[Haworth co-indexing entry note]: "Of Breasts and Men: Three Generations of Vampire Coupling." Schoenewolf, Gerald. Co-published simultaneously in *Journal of Couples Therapy* (The Haworth Press, Inc.) Vol. 8, No. 2, 1999, pp. 73-83; and: *Couples and Pregnancy: Welcome, Unwelcome, and In-Between* (ed: Barbara Jo Brothers) The Haworth Press, Inc., 1999, pp. 73-83. Single or multiple copies of this article are available for a fee from The Haworth Document Delivery Service [1-800-342-9678, 9:00 a.m. - 5:00 p.m. (EST). E-mail address: getinfo@haworthpressinc.com].

circumstances left him with a phobia about women's breasts. He could not stand them and he could not tolerate what they stood for–nurturing and intimacy. If there was any sucking to be done, it would have to be done on their necks, not their breasts, and the sucking would have violent consequences, as in the dream. He is one of a number of passive males I have treated who had such fantasies and dreams. All of them were involved with women who were much more aggressive than they were, whom they frustrated sexually and emotionally.

His relationship with his wife was a passive-aggressive struggle. The daily theme was one of frustration and counter-frustration. She wanted to have sex often and for long periods of time, whereas he was indifferent to it. She wanted to raise children, whereas he did not care one way or the other about marriage or children. She wanted to have long intimate talks with him, whereas he wanted to have long intimate talks with his computer. As the years of their relationship mounted, he had retreated further into passivity and she further into aggression. While in his dreams he sucked her blood, in real life he saw her as a vampire who was sucking his.

During the course of his individual treatment we were able to trace his passivity and his breast phobia to the deprivation he had undergone during the oral stage. The nature of the deprivation and aggression by his mother had caused him to repress his frustration and accompanying rage and to develop a passive character structure. Hence his passivity had an underlying aggressive undertow. Although he was badly in need of nurturing from a woman, he could not accept nurturing from his wife and in fact passively frustrated both her attempts to nurture and to be nurtured by him. At the same time, his passive-aggression aroused in his wife a type of response which I have earlier referred to as aggressive-passive (Schoenewolf, 1996). That is, she aggressed against him in such a way as to induce passivity and make him retreat even more into his shell, which gave her the excuse to criticize him all the more and achieve the secondary gain of displacing pent-up anger from her own childhood. This process served to reinforce each of their defensive postures and keep them stuck in a duel. In effect, he induced her to behave like his mother.

His relationship with his wife represented the third rendition in three generations of this kind of oral-sadistic coupling. During the course of his treatment, we found traces of it in the relationship of his mother and father, and his mother's mother and father. In each instance, the couples were apparently engaged in the same passive-aggressive duel. In each instance, a kind of vampire attitude permeated the relationship, so that instead of nurturing one another, each mate sucked life from the other. In each instance, the advent of pregnancy, childbirth, and nursing exacerbated the situation.

What finally broke the cycle of "vampire coupling" was that the wife of the dreamer of the vampire dream became pregnant, gave birth, and proceeded to somewhat blatantly suckle a girl child in front of her husband. His passive-aggression no longer worked, since his wife now had another object with which to satisfy her oral and emotional needs. Indeed, he not only felt powerless but also excluded (and, in a sense, cuckolded) by the nursing child. This eventually sent him into therapy, wherein he was able to work his way out of this syndrome and break a three-generation cycle.

FROM THE LITERATURE

In folklore, vampires were said to be ghosts of heretics, criminals, or madmen. They returned from the grave in the guise of monstrous bats to suck the blood of sleeping persons, who then became vampires themselves. The only way to kill them was to drive a wooden stake through their hearts. In Stoker's *Dracula* (1887), the vampire slept in a coffin by day and came out at night. Vampires have traditionally been male, and their victims have primarily been innocent, virginal females. The vampire myth, looked at analytically, would seem to correspond to the fantasies and dreams of dysfunctionally passive males, and may well be an outgrowth of such fantasies. Indeed, vampires are the epitome of passive males: they are so passive they are dead, and become revived only upon sucking living blood. They must kill others (turn them into vampires) in order to continue to live. In addition, through sucking the blood of innocent young women, they also attain super powers–they can only be killed in a certain proscribed way. This points to a grandiose, narcissistic component of such fantasies.

The vampire myth and dreams and fantasies that contain vampire themes have been attributed by psychological investigators to the oral-sadistic stage. Abraham writes of the vampire-like behavior of individuals whose breast-feeding was frustrated. He notes that such individuals always seem to be demanding something, and the nature of their demands has a quality of persistent sucking. Neither the facts nor reason can prevent their pleading and insisting. He notes that " . . . their behavior has an element of cruelty in it as well, which makes them something like vampires to other people" (1927, p. 401). The cruel sucking behavior of which he writes not only relates to the passive male, but might also have a link with the aggressive-passive females in the three generations of couples I am studying in this paper. He describes such people as alternately sucking like vampires and then giving out an "obstinate oral discharge." That is, they talk as a means of controlling and psychologically killing off their adversaries.

Klein was the first to draw attention to the significance of the "bad breast" in children's fantasies. She wrote of oral-sadistic fantasies of toddlers containing ideas that the child "gets possession of the contents of his mother's breast by sucking and scooping it out" (1932, p. 128). She describes an early stage of development "governed by the child's aggressive trends against its mother's body and in which its predominant wish is to rob her body of its contents and destroy it" (ibid.).

She goes on to explain that the feeling of emptiness in its body, which the child experiences as a result of lack of oral satisfaction, might be responsible for the fantasies of assault on the mother's body, since "it might give rise to phantasies of the mother's body being full of all the desired nourishment" (ibid.). Boys in particular harbor tremendous fear of the mother as castrator, and their attacks on the mother's body are also directed at their father's penis, which they imagine is inside their mother's body. "He is afraid of her as a person whose body contains his father's penis" (p. 131). Ideas about the phallic woman have their origin, according to Klein's research with little boys, during the oral-sadistic stage.

Freud (1910), in a study of Leonardo da Vinci, focused on the artist's memory of a vulture-like bird that came to him when he was an infant. According to the memory, while Leonardo was in his cradle, this threatening bird came down and opened the infant's mouth with its tail and struck him again and again with its tail. Freud contended that this memory was in fact a fantasy. The fantasy conceals a memory of being suckled at his mother's breast. The fact that in the fantasy the mother is replaced by the vulture-like bird–or perhaps a hawk, according to some (Andersen, 1994)–is an indication that the child experienced this suckling as something menacing.

Da Vinci was an illegimate child, which perhaps caused his mother to cling to him all the more. Freud speculates that this birth deprived him of a father's influence until his fifth year, and left him vulnerable to the "tender seductions of his mother," whose only solace he was. In his primitive fantasy, da Vinci saw this mother's nursing as aggressive and terrifying. At any rate, something happened during the nursing state to create in da Vinci a phobia of breasts. The memory or fantasy of da Vinci can be seen as evidence of trauma during the oral-sadistic stage. It seems to suggests a kind of oral rape.

Fenichel notes that "Oral-sadistic tendencies are often vampirelike in character" (1945, p. 489). He documents a case in which an infant was breast-fed for a year and a half, while living with a doting grandmother who spoiled him, and then was suddenly removed and forced to live with an excessively severe father. This childhood is somewhat similar to da Vinci's, with similar results. In Fenichel's case, the man became an extremely passive-dependent personality, who throughout his adulthood lived (sucked) on his father's money, who always felt his father had discriminated against him and was convined that life was unfair. He points out that the conflict between ingratiating submissiveness and an impulse violently to take what they think is theirs is characteristic of such types.

Socarides, writing of the dreams of passive males of what he calls the "perverse" variety, interprets that their inner stress stems, among other things, from the "threat of imminent destructive incorporation by the mother" (1980, p. 249). Spitz (1965), in a study of mothers and infants in a clinic for unwed mothers, details cases of what he calls "primary active rejection" by mothers who, due to their circumstances (being teenagers who were suddenly saddled with the responsibility for a child) had an extreme distaste for motherhood. He cites a case in which a mother stiffened and looked annoyed whenever she held her baby, and remarks, "During nursing the mother behaved as if her infant were completely alien to her and not a living being at all" (p. 211). Shengold (1979) has labeled a drastic form of anti-nurturing as "soul murder." According to him, the subject of such parenting is "robbed of his identity and of the ability to maintain authentic feelings. "Soul murder," he maintains, "remains effective if the capacity to think and to know has been sufficiently interfered with–by way of brainwashing" (p. 557). Others who have alluded to the kind of early deprivation that renders children passive include Ferenczi (1933), Laing (1971), Miller (1984), and Seinfield (1990).

Among family therapists, Satir (1967), wrote of marriages in which each partner needed the other to bolster his or her self-esteem. They chose a mate on the basis of the mate's capacity to elevate self esteem, and when that hope later fails the resulting feeling of loss and rejection is passed onto the children, who are treated as if they are the cause of the parents failure. Satir notes that this kind of dysfunctional family system often results in children who reject themselves. "A child needs to esteem himself in two areas: as a masterful person and as a sexual person" (p. 54). Obviously this did not happen with the subject of this study.

THREE GENERATIONS OF VAMPIRE COUPLING

John was about 30 years old at the time he had the dream reported at the beginning of this paper. He and Mary had been married for five years. As previously mentioned, their relationship had remain on a passive-aggressive level until Mary became pregnant. From the moment he found out she was pregnant, John began expressing vague feelings of annoyance and trepidation. He was not sure what he was annoyed or afraid of, until after the birth. When he caught sight of his wife breast-feeding their daughter, he discovered that what he was feeling was jealousy and rage. This jealousy and rage was brought on, first of all, by Mary's deliberate flaunting (so it seemed to him) of her nursing sessions, which he believed was her way of getting revenge for his years of frustration of her sexual and emotional needs. Second, it was aroused by a memory from the past, which had formerly been repressed, of his own oral frustration at the hands of his mother. This memory engendered a fear of reengulfment and, through the mechanism of projection, an irrational conviction that his wife's breasts were angry and dangerous things. The scene also bought back a later memory of witnessing his mother nursing his infant sister and feeling excluded from this intimacy, which induced a womb-envy that was the bedrock of his later envy of, and anger at, his wife's breasts and her capacity to nurse their daughter. This, in turn, later surfaced in his dreams.

John reported that his mother always preferred his younger sister and was hostile toward him on account of his being male. This seemed to be in part a response to frustrations she was experiencing with respect to his father, and in part due to traumas she had experienced in connection with her father (John's maternal grandfather). His mother continually complained about both men, but mostly about her husband, who would stay at work till late each night in order, she thought, to avoid her, and when he did come home he would be too sleepy to have sex, talk, or relate. Often his mother would scream at his father and the father would promise to reform, but he never would. In general the problems of John's mother and father trickled down and got displaced onto him through the manner in which his mother nursed him.

John reported that his mother had a problem with breast milk during the time she was nursing him and had to abruptly change to bottle-feeding, despite his vehement protests, and would put the bottle in a holder rather than holding him herself. This first trauma was later reinforced when he witnessed his mother breast-feeding his sister. Although he could not put it into words at the time, he felt that she had milk for his sister because she was a female, but none for him because he was male, and he resented it. When he wanted to join in on the action (she had an extra breast did she not?) she would shame him: "You're not a baby anymore. Run along and play."

John's mother had apparently flaunted her nursing of John and his sister in front of the father in an aggressive-passive way (aggression designed to induce passive rage in her husband). Instead of going into treatment as John had, the father stayed later at the office. Soon John's parents were separated, then divorced. Following the divorce, and for ten years after, until she remarried again, his mother did not allow his father to visit, even though the courts had ordered it. Nor did she allow his name to be spoken in the house.

John was forced to "swallow" everything: the oedipal guilt, the separation anxiety, the fear of maternal reengulfment, and the sibling jealousy. There was no soothing from his mother, nor a chance to ventilate or work through anything. Instead, he was made to feel that his feelings were wrong, stupid, or masculine. This constituted another layer of frustration added to the original layer of frustration during the oral stage, reinforcing the early repression.

He and his wife's relationship was almost a carbon copy of that of his mother and father. He treated Mary similarly to the way his father had treated his mother. He became passive-aggressive, fearing that his wife (his mother in the transference) would control and oppress him (suck his blood) rather than nurturing him. She was aggressive-passive, believing she had to constantly nag him and shame him in order to get any semblence of love or consideration from him. And so they remained at odds, both needing nurturing, each depriving the other of it.

In the sexual sphere, this manifested itself in her being grabby and of his being withholding. She would continually demand sex and complain that he did not satisfy her. He would perform sex as he might perform a duty like mowing the lawn (or, like a zombie mowing the lawn). She suffered from frigidity and blamed it on him. He suffered from premature ejaculation and blamed it on her. A huge sticking point of their sexual relations was his absolute refusal to ever kiss or suck her breasts. Almost weekly she would complain about this, and almost weekly he would continue to refuse.

John's mother's parents represented the third generation of oral-sadistic (vampire) coupling. For all I know it might have gone further and further back, but this is as far as we could trace it in therapy. From his mother's complaints about his father (John's grandfather), he deduced that this man too had been passive-aggressive, while his mother's mother had also been aggressive-passive, prone to temper tantrums. And once again, in this third generation, the birth of a child had apparently brought about a variation in the relationship; during the grandmother's pregnancy and for a year or so afterward, the grandfather had an affair with his secretary.

THE CLINICAL PICTURE

The man who became my patient was depleted of vitality and lived almost entirely in his dreams and fantasies. His fantasies were so important to him that for a long time he was reluctant to tell them to me or anybody. Indeed, the world of his fantasies was more real and more important to him than the real world. For the most part these fantasies were benign and bore no indication of the cruelty that would show up in his dreams at a later stage: trips to foreign planets where he became an heroic savior; inventions that made him famous; speeches before the United Nations that roused people to action. These fantasies—which had a Walter Mitty flavor—were indicative of his state of narcissism, which was almost at a delusional degree in the beginning of treatment.

The therapy relationship was a replica of his relationship with his wife and with people in general: passive-aggressive. In the beginning he was ingratiatingly submissive, giggling almost everytime he spoke. If I asked him, "What are you feeling right now?" he would respond, "I don't know," and giggle.

He dutifully brought in dreams, talked about his life, his work, his history, without any emotion except the giggle. At the same time, he had a great deal of problems paying me for sessions, and at one point there were ten bad checks in about twelve weeks.

Gradually, over several years, due to the working-through of the transference, his relationship with me changed into a more truly cooperative one, and the passive-aggression diminished. I encouraged him to confront his wife's demands rather than retreating into his world of fantasy, and his relationship with her began to change too, as well as his relationship with his parents. Toward the end of four years of therapy, he had the dream recounted at the beginning of this paper.

He had a number of dreams with vampire themes. In the first, recounted here, he was in an ambulance (a womb), where he injected a syringe (phallus) into a black woman (his sister, who in a reversal to what had actually occurred, became the "black sheep" of the family), so that she would die and he could live (be born). This may represent a wish that he might have prevented his mother's pregnancy. Later he does the same thing to his mother and her friends, siphoning off their blood so he could live. This perhaps represents another reversal of what he felt had been done to him in early childhood.

In another dream he was in a bus (another womb?) and touched the thumb of the woman sitting next to him with his thumb (her phallus with his?) causing her to tremble and die. In yet a third dream he was swimming in a rough sea, and there was a wall separating the sea from the land, and the wall had a long tunnel in it. To get to the tunnel (mother's womb), he had to walk on the backs of several female swimmers ahead of him (his sister and her friends), causing them to drown. Finally he made it to the tunnel.

Aside from the vampire motif, the dreams may be seen to have other layers of meaning. The first two dreams, in which he injected a syringe into a woman's neck and touched another's thumb with his thumb, may suggest that he saw himself as possessing a poisonous phallus. This might represent incestuous feelings or it could be an indication of womb envy or an introjection of his mother's and sister's scorn of his masculinity. In one dream he was out in a rough sea and a wall separated him from land. This may denote his feeling of being excluded by women–being tossed out to sea–or separated from his mother's womb. In the first dream, where the ambulance perhaps symbolizes the womb, he is apparently still-born. (He often verbalized the feeling that his birth wasn't wanted.) Giving the women in the dreams two or three penises may be his way of assuaging his castration fear. There are undoubtedly other meanings I haven't covered, but these seem most relevant to this study.

I considered these dreams to be significant signposts in his therapy. They were sharper, and more emotionally tinged than earlier dreams, indicating to me that previously taboo material about the extent of his sexual frustration and aggression was coming to the surface. By being held up in relief, the dreams seemed to clearly show the oral-sadistic underpinning of his personality.

Prior to these vampire dreams, he had not been able to get in touch with his anger. The only person toward whom he could feel anger was his father, who happened to be the only person his mother allowed him to feel anger towards. He was misled by the mother into believing that the father had abandoned him and had chosen not to visit him. In actuality, the mother refused to allow his visits, but the father passively accepted this refusal without putting up a legal fight. Hence John, in identification with his mother, would often express resentment toward his father: "If only he had not left, things would have been different." In addition, through a negative identification with his father, he saw both himself and his father as a bad, somewhat pathetic figures.

Along with the emergence of the dreams came a breakage of the repression of his feelings. He began to express more anger at his mother, his wife, and me. Much of the early work of therapy consisted in helping him individuate and separate from his mother. During this phase, he began to drop the submissive, giggly false self and to verbalize the distrust and anger underneath. For a time he treated me as though I were going to latch onto him, make him totally dependent on me, and suck his blood (the mother transference). He became suddenly concerned about the fee, whereas previously he had paid no attention to it. He expressed the view that I was financially and emotionally exploiting him, that my interpretations were hostile reproaches, and that the only reason I wished to keep him in therapy was to gratify myself at his expense. By verbalizing these things and analyzing them, he was able to pull himself out of the passive-aggressive, oral-sadistic defensive mode.

He was then able to explore how the same dynamics had come into play in his relationship with his wife, and to reach this same state of aliveness and realness with her. He first expressed to me, then to her, his fears of her sucking his blood, and underneath this an even bigger fear of allowing himself to be nurtured by her (and become dependent and devoured by her). As he worked through this material, his wife was able to let go of her own aggressive-passive mode. Their relationship became more real, their relationship with their daughter became more real and their parenting became more a partnering, give-and-take venture rather than a ritual of marital war. In essence I was able to do couples therapy by working with one member directly and the other indirectly.

CONCLUSION

This study focused on how certain modes of relating are passed on from generation to generation. In this case, as I reconstructed the patient's history,

I encountered three renditions of a similar pattern of relating, which I term "vampire coupling" because of its oral-sadistic nature. These relationships were characterized by a passive-aggressive struggle in which each member of the couple frustrated the other's oral needs for nurturing.

It appears this kind of coupling results in childrearing that tends to pass onto children the parents' inherent frustration and discontentment. That is to say, orally-deprived, sadistic parents tend to produce orally-deprived, sadistic children. The early psychoanalytic writings on oral sadism by Freud, Klein, and Abraham allude to the vampire-like behavior of individuals who have developed certain types of fixations in the oral stage and provide some theoretical base for understanding extreme forms of orality. However, these early analysts were more concerned with drive theory and did not adequately understand the significance of maternal aggression, paternal passivity, and its impact on the child's fantasies and subsequent development. I have tried in this paper to fill in this gap as best I could, showing the possible results of a particular kind of oral deprivation and sadism.

Regarding the vampire myth, it would seem to be an outcome of the passive, perhaps schizoid, fantasies and dreams of both males and females. The fact that it has been present in Western culture since Medieval times, if not before, shows that it may be a universal phenomenon that serves as a grandiose compensation for the collective fears of humanity–fears related to castration and oral frustration and reengulfment. The myth is also perhaps an expression of narcissistic rage. This myth, like vampire dreams, affords a symbolic enactment of the some of humankind's collective fears, harking back to early oral deprivation. It may serve to dissipate some of that rage, just as dreams serve to dissipate the accumulated frustrations of the day. As such, it is a close relative of other similar myths about witches, Frankensteins, dragons, and werewolves.

REFERENCES

Abraham, K. (1927). *Selected Papers on Psycho-Analysis.* New York: Brunner/Mazel, 19791.

Anderson, W. (1994). Leonardo da Vinci and the slip that fooled almost everybody. *Psychoanalysis and Contemporary Thought,* 17-483-515.

Fenichel, O. (1945). *The Psychoanalytic Theory of Neurosis.* New York: Norton.

Ferenczi, S. (1933). Confusion of tongue between adults and the child. In *Further Contributions to the Theory and Technique of Psycho-Analysis,* pp. 126-147. New York: Brunner/Mazel, 1980.

Freud, S. (1910). Leonardo da Vinci and a memory of his childhood. *Standard Edition,* 11:59-138.

Klein, M. (1932). *The Psychoanalysis of Children.* New York: Delacorte Press, 1975.

Laing, R. D. (1971). *The Politics of the Family.* Harmondsworth, England: Penguin Books.

Miller, A. (1984). *For Your Own Good: The Hidden Cruelty in Childhood and the Roots of Violence*. New York: Farrar, Straus & Girous.

Schoenewolf, G. (1996). *The Couple Who Fell in Hate*. Northvale, NJ: Jason Aronson.

Seinfeld, J. (1990). *The Bad Object*. Northvale, NJ: Jason Aronson.

Satir, V. (1967). *Conjoint Family Therapy*, Revised Edition. Palo Alto, CA: Science and Behavior Books.

Shengold, L. L. (1979). Child abuse and deprivation: soul murder. *Journal of the American Psychoanalytic Association*, 17:533-560.

Socarides, C. (1980). A unitary theory of sexual perversions. In *On Sexuality*, ed. by T. B. Karasu and C. W. Socarides, pp. 161-188. New York: International Universities Press.

Spitz, R. (1965). *The First Year of Life*. New York: International Universities Press.

Stoker, B. (1887). *Dracula*. London: Hogarth.

Comment:
"Of Breasts and Men" . . .
and Use of Psychoanalytic Theory

Barbara Jo Brothers

SUMMARY. Comment on Schoenewolf's preceding article, "Of Breasts and Men" and discussion of transcriptions of an interview with Virginia Satir on the shortcomings of psychoanalytic theory, including excerpts from "Virginia Satir," written by Barbara Jo Brothers to be included in *Circle of Influence*, edited by Melvin Suhd. *[Article copies available for a fee from The Haworth Document Delivery Service: 1-800-342-9678. E-mail address: getinfo@haworthpressinc.com <Website: http://www. haworthpressinc.com>]*

KEYWORDS. Satir, psychoanalytic theory, pathologizing

This article seems, in some way, to go for the jugular on an emotional level, judging from the wildly disparate responses from *Journal of Couples Therapy* reviewers.

The first reviewer declined to rate the article at all, suggesting that it be sent to a more analytically oriented person, expressing concern about sexism in the article. That reviewer wanted to know, for example, how is the author defining "aggressive women"? And, "What would DaVinci have done without his mother?"

The next reviewer responded:

> The secondary title and opening paragraphs of this paper lead me to expect a horror movie, with violence and sex mixed together in a

---

Excerpts from "Virginia Satir" in *Circle of Influence* are printed with permission of Science & Behavior Books, Mountain View, CA.

[Haworth co-indexing entry note]: "Comment: 'Of Breasts and Men' . . . and Use of Psychoanalytic Theory." Brothers, Barbara Jo. Co-published simultaneously in *Journal of Couples Therapy* (The Haworth Press, Inc.) Vol. 8, No. 2, 1999, pp. 85-89; and: *Couples and Pregnancy: Welcome, Unwelcome, and In-Between* (ed: Barbara Jo Brothers) The Haworth Press, Inc., 1999, pp. 85-89.

package. Later the author treats the material in a slightly more scholarly and professional manner. In several places he refers to a study, technically this is a case *study* or, better, a case history.

I object to statements implying that people have no choice about their feelings and behaviors, i.e., she "makes" him, or oral deprivation "causes" this. It is just poor conceptualization.

Neither the patient nor his wife are presented as having any positive strengths. The patient, at least, had the resources to seek therapy and hang in there with both therapist and wife while dealing with quite difficult feelings. There is not a very clear differentiation between the patient's and the therapist's fantasies. The therapy process is not described.

Marilyn Yalom's new book, *A History of the Breast*, might be of interest; she has a chapter on the psychoanalytic view of the breast that quotes some of the same material.

As an aside, Spitz's data on anaclitic depression has been found to have been fraudulent.

The paper might be more appropriate in a psychoanalytically oriented journal, but I doubt it contributes anything new to the field. In any event, this type of "wild" analytic presentation has contributed greatly to the criticism of psychoanalysis and to a lack of appreciation of what good analytic thinking and treatment can contribute.

In sum, I cannot recommend it be published in the *Journal of Couples Therapy.*

In contrast, the third writes:

> Very well-written, creative and interesting article–showing complexity in individuals and how pathology becomes mutuality in couples. It combines clinical/dream material with solid psychoanalytic theory–both being used to demonstrate a not-uncommon couples issue.
>
> It is also somewhat of a change from most *Journal of Couples Therapy* articles, drawing more on psychoanalytic theory–should be interesting to see reader's response.
>
> I liked it.

This reviewer gave it a 9/10 to the second reviewer's 2. The fourth reviewer, who also gave a 2 rating, says:

> I found the article interesting and thought provoking. In spite of my enjoyment, I vote that we *not* publish it. I base my decision that we not publish it on my opinion that it is not a good fit for the *Journal of Couples Therapy*. I suggest that the author send this article to a psycho-

analytically-oriented journal and get good psychoanalytic editorial input. It has possibilities, but needs some more careful bridging with psychoanalytic theory.

Maybe it is because I live in Ann Rice's* hometown and am inured to vampires. Against the advice of three editorial board members, I chose to publish Schoenewolf's article.

As I read "Of Breasts and Men," I noted the example couple reminded me of my parents. The author was striking familiar chords; these were dynamics I have seen in action. My own aversion to psychoanalytic theory notwithstanding, I find it possible to receive his psychoanalytic language simply as dramatic metaphor, a symbolic representation of behavior, even if demeaning in tone.

However, for the most part, I agree with the reviewers' implied objections to thinking in such disparaging terms about one's patients and in describing them accordingly. A number of years ago, I held an interview with Virginia Satir (1916-1988) in which she voiced her reservations about an exclusively psychoanalytic orientation, in spite of her respect for Freud and his work.

From *Circle of Influence*:

BJB: What kind of personal therapy did you get?

VS: I went through a full psychoanalysis and actually the main things never got touched. That was another thing, I had a good analyst from an analytic point of view but the things that were really basic to me, really troubling me, never got touched because psychoanalysis is limited in its ability to handle things. When I was through with it I said to myself, "There's gotta be more than this." Because, actually, I see the whole thing of psychoanalysis as a rather pessimistic thing about the hopefulness in people. While I have a great deal of respect for Freud as someone who opened the barriers, I don't consider that Freud and psychoanalysis have that much in common, because he was somebody who was always moving ahead and psychoanalysis got frozen in time by his followers.

I went into analysis, after I had already finished the school of social work in the late 1940s, because I was having some rather serious physical problems. The physicians told me, "This is not a physical problem; it's a psychological problem." So the only thing I knew to do, being in a city and in work that was so psychiatrically oriented, was to get psychoanalyzed; so that's what I did. It helped the physical things, but it didn't really remove the basic things behind them. So I felt even

---

*Rice, A. (1977). *Interview with the vampire*. New York: Ballentine Books.

more freedom then to look to see what else there was. I didn't see
anything else, so I started looking at me. (1983, p. 50)

. . . [Thus] Virginia began her part in the inventive creation of a new mode
of psychotherapy: including the whole family in simultaneous treatment. She
called this *conjoint family therapy.*

While she created this new modality partially as a result of the experimen-
tal attitude that characterized all her work, she was also on a conscious quest
to improve on psychoanalysis, which was the only kind of therapy in practice
then. She had found it wanting. Her own analysis had failed to help her
identify or address vital issues, and she was disillusioned about the derogato-
ry attitude inherent in the analytic mode. These were motivating factors for
her creation of her comprehensive, growth-based model.

Inventing family therapy meant venturing into the whole system from
which a person emerges. By asking the entire family to attend sessions,
Virginia could observe people's whole context and intervene in any aspect of
it. She could actually watch (rather than just hear about) the family dynamics:
how the behavior of one family member affected the rest. All in all, through
working with the entire family, she found herself able to promote the emerging personhood of parent and child alike.

Her insights into what would be therapeutically useful were by no means
always the result of a series of happy accidents, as she would sometimes
present it. They were the product of her relentless search for knowledge–for
salient information on human behavior–and of her remarkable genius for
synthesis . . .

By 1951 she had seen her first family:

I went into private practice in 1951, and, in 1951 in Chicago, of course,
everything was completely psychoanalytic. I got the people that nobody
else wanted. I knew the psychoanalytic method wasn't going to work so
I was from scratch. Of course, you can't always be from scratch because you're influenced by things, but one thing I didn't do was that I
never followed the dictates of the psychoanalytic idea that you had to
be aloof from your patients. I really violated a great many things in that
regard. I was still looking for something more. There had to be something more and so that's kind of how that all started. And then it just
evolved from there. I'm still looking. (Satir in Brothers, 1983, p. 50)

One of those "violations" was seeing the client's family. In those heavily
psychoanalytic days, this was considered a serious breach of good therapy.
This "transgression," now well known, was the beginning of her work with
families. Today, of course, the mental health field actively prescribes what

was once forbidden–after the pioneering work done by Virginia Satir, Murray Bowen, and Don Jackson.

> . . . It was this willingness to depart from the norm that paved the way for Virginia's brilliant insights into the critical relationship between self-esteem and communication. With two clients in the consulting room, the therapist can observe interaction as well as participate. Virginia's work thus assumed that all human experience is relational. Individual dynamics could almost be said to be an illusion, as no human being ever functions as utterly separate from other human beings. Our young do not scramble alone to the sea like young turtles. Even the monk in contemplation in the desert still carries internalized dialogue from his own family of origin. Any psychological theory explaining the human animal must take into account the intense interactional factor. Virginia, whose mind was never limited by practices currently in vogue, understood this. [in press]

In essence, Virginia Satir's substantial contribution to the invention of family therapy was born partially of her personal experience with the shortcomings of the theory that was the only show in town at the time. Rather than negating Freud's work, she seemed to see herself as extending it, adding what had been missing.

This volume begins with Virginia Satir's belief in the importance of celebrating differences as an aspect of uniqueness. In that spirit, we include "Of Breasts and Men." While departing from the usual tone of the *Journal of Couples Therapy,* Schoenewolf's article does provide a view of a certain form of toxic interaction between a couple. Although somewhat jarring to those of us who are not comfortable with the "pathologizing" aspects of psychoanalytic terminology, there is merit to remaining open to such differing viewpoints and languages. Otherwise, babies may be thrown out with bathwater and diamonds may be discarded with coal dust.

REFERENCES

Brothers, B. J. (1983). Virginia Satir: Past to present. *Voices: The Art and Science of Psychotherapy, 18:* (Win.):48-56.
Brothers, B.J. Virginia Satir. In Melvin Suhd (Ed.) *Circle of Influence.* Mountain View, Calif: Science and Behavior Books. [in press]
Rice, A. (1977). *Interview with the vampire.* New York: Ballentine Books.

Index

Abortion choice. *See also*
  Post-abortion grief
  couple systems and, 37,39
  defined, 62
  effect on men, 61
  grieving and
    case history, 46-47
  male response to
    case history, 62-64
  marital pregnancy and
    case history (1), 43-45
    case history (2), 45-47
  therapist's role in management of,
    48
Abuse. *See* Sexual abuse (childhood)
Activators *versus* creators Virginia
    Satir and, 1-2
Actualization
  goals in experiential psychotherapy,
    21-22
Adoption choice
  concealed
    couple systems and, 37
  premarital pregnancy and case
    history, 39-42
  therapist's role in management of,
    48
Aggressive-passive behavior
  described, 74
  vampire-coupling mode of relating
    and, 79-80
Anniversary dates
  perinatal loss and, 54
Anti-nurturing
  effect on children, 77
Anticipation. *See* Planning
Avanta Process Community Meetings
  excerpts from transcripts
    1982 meeting, 3-4

1993 Meeting, 4
August 1981 meeting, 2-3
Virginia Satir's lectures and, 1-2

Bereavement Services/RTS, 51
Biomedical perspective
  infertility and, 21
Biomedical treatment
  for infertility, 18-19
Birth of child
  as a result of sexual intercourse, 8
  developmental stage of parent and,
    8
  psychological effects on parents'
    intimacy, 7,8
Breast feeding, effect of frustration of,
    75,77
Breasts
  bad breast fantasies in children,
    75-76
  phobia
    case history, 73-74
  psychoanalytic view of, 86
  vampire-coupling and, 77-78

Child-care experiences
  activating life force and, 4
  activation implications for, 1
  first child
    compared with second or
      subsequent children, 13-14
Childbirth
  therapists' understanding of issues
    of, 14
Children
  death of, devastation of couple
    system and, 38